Positive Options for Hiatus Hernia

About the Author

Dr. Tom Smith spent six years in general practice and seven years in medical research before taking up writing full time in 1977. He writes regularly for medical journals and magazines; contributes frequently to the Scottish *Carrick Gazette*, the *Galloway Gazette*, and the *Stornoway Gazette*; broadcasts regularly on health matters on BBC Radio Scotland; and won the Third Prize in the British Medical Journalists Awards for 2000 for an essay he wrote for *The Herald*. He is the author of the books *Living with High Blood Pressure*, *Coping with Strokes*, *Coping with Bronchitis and Emphysema*, *Heart Attacks: Prevent and Survive*, *Living with Angina*, and *Coping with Stomach Ulcers* (all published in the U.K. by Sheldon Press) and also writes and updates clinician's manuals on the treatment of disease for Science Press in London. He still maintains part-time general practice in southwest Scotland. He is married and has two married children and five grandchildren.

D1005133

Ordering

Trade bookstores in the U.S. and Canada please contact:

Publishers Group West
1700 Fourth Street, Berkeley CA 94710
Phone: (800) 788-3123   Fax: (510) 528-3444

Hunter House books are available at bulk discounts for textbook course adoptions; to qualifying community, healthcare, and government organizations; and for special promotions and fund-raising. For details please contact:

Special Sales Department
Hunter House Inc., PO Box 2914, Alameda CA 94501-0914
Phone: (510) 865-5282   Fax: (510) 865-4295
E-mail: ordering@hunterhouse.com

Individuals can order our books from most bookstores or by calling toll-free:
(800) 266-5592

Positive Options

for

HIATUS HERNIA

Self-Help and Treatment

Tom Smith, M.D.

Hunter House
PUBLISHERS

Hunter House Inc., Publishers
PO Box 2914
Alameda CA 94501-0914

First published in Great Britain in 1997 by
Sheldon Press, SPCK, Marylebone Road, London NW1 4DU

Library of Congress Cataloging-in-Publication Data

Smith, Tom, Dr.
Positive options for hiatus hernia: self-help and treatment/Tom Smith.
    p. cm
Includes Index.
ISBN 0-89793-318-4 (pb.) -- ISBN 0-89793-319-2 (cl.)
    1. Hiatal hernia--popular works. 2. Hiatal hernia--Treatment--
Popular works. 3. Self-care, Health. I. Title.
RC815.7 .S596 2001
617.5'59--dc21   00-054687

Project Credits

Cover Design: *osprey*design
Book Production: Hunter House
Copy Editor: Kelley Blewster
Proofreader: John David Marion
Indexer: Kathy Tally-Jones
Acquisitions Editor: Jeanne Brondino
Associate Editor: Alexandra Mummery
Editorial/Production Assistant: Melissa Millar
Publicity Manager: Sarah Frederick
Marketing Assistant: Earlita Chenault
Administrator: Theresa Nelson
Customer Service Manager: Christina Sverdrup
Order Fulfillment: Joel Irons
Publisher: Kiran S. Rana

RC
815.7
.5596
2001

Printed and Bound by Publishers Press, Salt Lake City, Utah

Manufactured in the United States of America
9 8 7 6 5 4 3 2 1   First Edition   01 02 03 04 05

Contents

Important Note

The material in this book is intended to provide a review of information regarding coping with hiatus hernia. Every effort has been made to provide accurate and dependable information. The contents of this book have been compiled through professional research and in consultation with medical professionals. However, health care professionals have differing opinions, and advances in medical and scientific research are made very quickly, so some of the information may become outdated.

Therefore, the publisher, authors, editors, and professionals quoted in the book cannot be held responsible for any error, omission, or outdated material. The authors and publisher assume no responsibility for any outcome of applying the information in this book in a program of self-care or under the care of a licensed practitioner. If you have questions concerning your nutrition or diet, or about the application of the information described in this book, consult a qualified health care professional.

Introduction

To have opened this book, you obviously found the title of interest. You may already know you have a hiatus hernia. Or you have heard or read about hiatus hernia and think it's possible that you have one, because your symptoms fit. If so, this book is for you. If you know your diagnosis, it will help you understand it more. If you think you may have the condition, the book will guide you through how a diagnosis may be made or ruled out. In either case, it will describe not only what your medical team can do for you, but, just as important, how you can help yourself to overcome your symptoms and the hernia itself.

You may call your symptoms "indigestion," "dyspepsia," "heartburn," or "an upset stomach." You may have been taking over-the-counter medicines for them for years, easing the symptoms, but never curing them. You are not alone. You are following a tradition that has endured for centuries. No home medicine cabinet is without medicines for indigestion, and particularly for heartburn—the fiery pain felt in the center of the chest. "Stomach" medicines take up the biggest section of any pharmacy. We have all had to take them at some time, and approximately one-third to one-half of the adult population takes them every day, to treat or prevent discomfort. Medication for heartburn and indigestion has become normal, rather than unusual.

People who take these medications often assume that the

cause of their symptoms is a sensitive stomach or an allergy, or even a stomach ulcer. They may even blame the food, so they avoid fries or any other food that they ate immediately before the symptoms arose. It is easy to assume that a particular food has a special effect on the stomach, when in fact there is strong evidence that the stomach is a very tolerant organ. A normal stomach allows us to widen enormously the range of foods we can eat without a moment's complaint or thought.

So why do so many people take indigestion remedies so often? For some there may be an element of gastritis—inflammation of the stomach. A few will have an ulcer. But for many more the true cause is a hiatus hernia (also called hiatal hernia).

This book is about hiatus hernias. It explains simply what they are, why they cause certain symptoms, how the symptoms can be relieved, and how people with hiatus hernias can live a normal life—without constant problems. A hiatus hernia is not a complicated condition, and if it is kept under control, it can be so easy to live with that it can almost be forgotten. But it does demand attention to lifestyle, as well as to its medical management and treatment. And for some people it may mean surgery.

Positive Options for Hiatus Hernia covers all aspects of the care of people with a hiatus hernia. It is meant for sufferers and for their partners and caregivers. It is based on the principle that if you, as a patient, know why you are asked to do (or not do) something, you will find it easier to comply with the advice. You will learn why it is better not to take the risk of bending over or lying flat, and you will learn when new symptoms should force you to see your doctor rather than treat yourself. It will also help you to recognize when your symptoms are *not* likely to be due to your hernia, but may be caused by something else. Hiatus hernia often causes chest pain, but so do heart and lung problems, and there may be a time when you need to know the difference—which is why I have devoted a chapter to sorting out these symptoms.

However, this is not a book to cause concern or worry; in fact it is just the reverse. Its tone is upbeat—positively optimistic—

because there are many ways in which the symptoms of a hiatus hernia can be minimized and its complications prevented, and most of them are under your own control. Hiatus hernia is a condition whose outcome, for the vast majority of people, depends almost entirely on themselves.

Of course, medical and sometimes surgical treatment does help, and for a few these are crucial. But if you can face up to the demands (in most cases they are pleasures) of a new lifestyle, you will almost certainly relieve your own symptoms and avoid the need for a specialist or hospital care.

Hiatus hernia affects all ages and both sexes. You may recognize yourself among the case histories in chapter 1. If so, please read on.

Chapter 1

A Few Fellow-Sufferers

This chapter contains a few case histories of hiatus hernia sufferers. They are all typical of the people who suffer from the complaint, though their symptoms differ widely. So if you don't relate to the first story, read on; you will probably see yourself in one of the others. And don't worry if you don't immediately understand all the details of the stories or the terms used. You'll find them explained in later chapters and in the glossary at the end of the book.

Mary's Story

Mary was fifty-eight when she first visited her doctor. Since her children had left home (she had been a full-time homemaker) and her life had become less hectic, she had put on a few pounds, so she had what is politely called a matronly figure. She was about five feet three inches tall and weighed more than 165 pounds.

Her "indigestion" symptoms had started about four years earlier. At first, she'd felt a sharp, raw pain in the center of her chest, with an occasional sour taste in the mouth that came on shortly after meals (or even a cup of tea), particularly when she was putting up her feet. She noticed, too, that the symptoms came on when she bent down, either to get things from beneath the kitchen counter or when she was weeding the garden.

She assumed that all this had to do with her increased weight or her age, or even with the fact that she had started to wear a support girdle—so she decided not to bother her doctor and instead treated herself. She started taking indigestion pills—antacids such as Rolaids™—and, at first, thought no more of her symptoms.

For the first few months, the antacids always eased her symptoms. In fact, they did so very quickly, far faster than she might have expected if the problem were inside her stomach—and that might have given her a clue that the problem was farther up, in her *esophagus* (the tube leading from the throat to the stomach).

However, this honeymoon period did not last. Gradually she found herself taking antacids every day. The pain lasted longer, came on more often, and was spreading farther up into her chest. To ease it, she started to drink copious amounts of milk and to eat cookies and crackers, which did nothing to help her weight problem. The character of her pain, too, had changed. It was by now clearly recognizable as heartburn—a burning sensation that she felt in a vertical line down the middle of her chest.

Even this was not enough to send her to the doctor. She assumed that heartburn was a common complaint that could be dealt with by over-the-counter medicines, and not the sort of problem with which to bother her doctor. So she continued self-treating with antacids and with servings of milk and cookies.

Two further developments finally brought her to her senses—and to the doctor's office. The first was a persistent, dull ache right in the center of her chest, just behind the inverted V at the lower end of her breastbone. It never seemed to go away completely, and sometimes it woke her at night. The second development was less regular but just as worrisome. The sour taste in the mouth had not only become much more frequent, but it had grown worse. She found her mouth filling with sour, watery material that had apparently welled up from her stomach (a substance known as *waterbrash*). It was sometimes so bad that it made her choke. Along with this, she found that she could no longer lie flat in bed at night, particularly if she lay on her right side. This invariably produced the waterbrash, and occasionally her mouth filled with the food that she had eaten an hour or so before. This happened one night in her sleep, and she awoke terrified—literally drowning on a mouthful of semidigested milk.

The next morning, in something approaching a panic, she saw her doctor, who had no difficulty making the diagnosis of a sliding hiatus hernia (see chapter 3), but who would have preferred knowing about it at a much earlier stage! Then her treatment would have been easier, and there would have been much less damage to reverse.

Eve's Story

Eve was forty when she noticed her first symptoms. Married with teenage children, Eve was an only daughter whose father, in the later stages of Alzheimer's disease, had recently moved in with her. A worrier at the best of times, Eve's stress after her father moved in became huge, and she was in no doubt that this was a direct cause of her symptoms.

However, her hernia did not show itself in pain or waterbrash. Instead, she had what she described as discomfort—a feeling that the food she had swallowed had not gone all the way into her stomach, but had stuck somewhere in the middle of her chest. Each time she ate, once she felt the sensation, she stopped eating, so meals became a real trial for her. There were times when she could not eat any solid food—indeed, was frightened of doing so, in case it stuck. So she tended to eat only semisolid foods and liquids, believing that they would go down more easily. As they tended to be minced meats and milky puddings, she started to put on weight.

Quite the opposite of Mary's case, however, she found that lying down actually helped her symptoms. Resting, when she could grab a minute, always seemed to allow something inside her to relax and let the food slide into the stomach. Her symptoms never started when she was in bed, and she never had a burning sensation or the flow of waterbrash into her mouth.

Her doctor at the time, worried about the symptom of food sticking in her chest, arranged for a barium-swallow X-ray examination, which showed a small hiatus hernia. This surprised him, as he was looking for other conditions more likely to produce the symptoms of blockage—the main one in women of Eve's age being *achalasia*, in which the lower end of the esophagus goes into spasm (a form of cramp), which eases with rest. But the barium showed quite clearly a rolling hiatus hernia, so he advised her on that basis. (Achalasia and the different types of hiatus hernia are explained in more detail in chapter 3, along with other conditions with which hiatus hernia can be confused.)

After her father died, and the main source of her stress had gone, her symptoms stopped. For twenty years, they did not return. Last year, Eve—now sixty years old and a healthy woman—developed a severe attack of shingles. Unfortunately, she first noticed the rash, which ran around the right side of her chest over her breast, at midday on a Saturday. Being considerate, she did not want to disturb her doctor on the weekend, so she treated herself until Monday morning with calamine lotion.

This was a mistake; it is vital that shingles are treated within the first thirty-six hours (preferably twenty-four hours) with the antiviral drug acyclovir (Zovirax). Acyclovir damps down the eruption, greatly eases the pain, and, most important, helps the patient avoid the sometimes very severe postshingles pain in the scarred area of skin left by the acute attack.

By Monday, Eve's shingles were a mess. A thick band of pustules and inflamed skin extended from the spine to the breastbone on the right side of her chest, and she was in severe pain and considerable distress. At this point, her hiatus hernia symptoms returned. Once again, eating produced a feeling of blockage. She had to confine her eating to porridge, soup, and custard, as nothing solid would go down. No amount of swallowing, she felt, would "push the food down." One crucial symptom was the pressing desire to belch. She had the ever-present feeling that there was gas in her chest or upper stomach and that she would get relief if only she could bring it up. But she found it impossible to do so. She thought that liquid antacids might help, so she scoured the drugstore for the best—but none helped her. Changing her body position did not help either. She spent hours rolling around in her chair or bed trying to find a position to give her relief from the gas or the "blockage," but it was all in vain.

Her doctor was convinced that the painkillers she was taking for the shingles had stimulated the return of the hernia symptoms. He therefore prescribed a drug to reduce any irritation in the stomach, while continuing with the painkillers. She gradually recovered from both the pain and the hernia symptoms, but it took her more than four months to feel confident enough to eat solid foods again.

Six months after the onset of the shingles attack, she is back to her normal self. She still tends to avoid lumpy foods (she makes sure she chews everything thoroughly before swallowing) and has gotten into the habit of eating several small meals a day, rather than three larger meals, because she feels uncomfortable with a full stomach. She avoids bending down—but only because she has heard that it is not good for a hiatus hernia, not because bending has ever bothered her. She no longer takes any medication and is doing well.

Harry's Story

Harry is sixty-eight and a retired electrician. His symptoms started when he was in his early fifties—with hiccups! They would come on late at night, in bed, just before he dropped off to sleep. He noticed that they were more likely to start if he'd eaten sweets, ice cream, or chocolate just before going to bed (he admitted to having a very sweet tooth). At the same time he felt what he described as discomfort (it wasn't painful or burning) in the upper middle region of his stomach, and a bloated feeling deep in his chest, as if gases were trapped inside it. Like Eve, at times like this he desperately wanted to belch, but couldn't. He assumed that this was just a reaction to eating too many sweet things and changed his late-evening habits. He took a glass of warm milk instead, which helped a little. Even then, the hiccups sometimes occurred when he lay down flat in bed. The only way to relieve them was to get up and walk around or sit up and read. Using extra pillows in bed helped, too. Being propped up at an angle of around 45 degrees kept the symptoms at bay and seemed to prevent the hiccups. After a few restless nights he became more used to sleeping in that position.

Ten years ago, things changed. While at work one day, crawling around under the floorboards of a house he was rewiring, Harry developed a severe pain in the center of his chest, felt very sick, and broke out into a cold, clammy sweat. A doctor was called, and Harry was admitted to the hospital with a suspected heart attack.

However, the hospital tests showed that these new symptoms were actually caused by an inflamed gallbladder, which was full of gallstones. It was assumed that his other symptoms were also related to his gallbladder disease, so when the gallbladder was removed a few weeks later, Harry expected his hiccups and discomfort to disappear. They didn't.

While the surgeons were removing his gallbladder, they checked on his diaphragm and confirmed that he had a hiatus hernia. However, they considered it not serious enough for a surgical repair and left it as it was.

Since then, Harry has been careful. He has had no recurrence of his gallbladder symptoms, though occasionally he still experiences evening hiccups and discomfort. But if he avoids bending over and eating anything after around 8:00 P.M., he remains relatively symptom-free. Recently he has been suffering the odd bout of heartburn, for which he takes one tablet of ranitidine (Zantac) a day, and that seems to help.

Two other changes in his life may also have contributed to his improvement. First, now that he has retired, he no longer must crawl around in confined spaces or lie on a floor with head and chest down a hole, working with electrical wiring. That must be about the worst occupation for anyone with a hiatus hernia! The other is that he has stopped smoking. He is living proof that someone can stop smoking after forty years and feel much the better for it. Doing so will certainly have done his stomach and hiatus hernia a power of good, as well, of course, as his lungs, heart, and blood vessels.

And now that he has retired, he has taken up golf. That keeps him fit, and with the exercise he has shed about twenty-eight pounds. The weight loss, too, may have improved the state of his hernia. He did think of taking up bowling, but was strongly advised against it; bowling is no game for anyone with a hiatus hernia.

Harry illustrates an important point. One in every five people with hiatus hernia has another related illness. The list includes duodenal and gastric ulcers, gallstones, and coronary heart disease, so even if a hiatus hernia has shown up in an X-ray (as in Eve's and Mary's cases) or has been seen during surgery (as in Harry's case), it should never be assumed that any symptoms around the upper stomach and chest are due to the hernia. That pain in the chest could be angina or a heart attack, and a pain in the upper stomach could be from an ulcer or gallstones. So if new symptoms arise, and they don't go away with the usual treatment, or if they are worse than usual, don't hesitate to seek urgent advice. It can often be difficult to distinguish between the pain of hiatus hernia and that of heart attack, but one thing is sure—taking an antacid usually eases hiatus hernia pain very quickly. It will make not a bit of difference to heart pain.

James's Story

James, at fifty, was a fairly stubborn man. A schoolteacher, he had no use for doctors and felt that he could look after himself very well without them. That may have been true when he was younger, but he had a failing that was nearly the death of him. He enjoyed his "little drink" in the evenings. It varied from a scalding hot cup of tea to a neat whisky, neither of which was compatible with his hiatus hernia, which he had treated by himself for many years.

He had started to experience mild heartburn in his late thirties. It was worse just after a meal—which for James, who lived on his own, was usually something quick he fried up himself—so he always kept a bottle of his favorite antacid mixture beside the kitchen sink. A day never passed without a swig from his white antacid bottle.

As the years passed, however, the symptoms worsened. With every meal, he experienced a deep-seated pain behind the lower half of his breastbone, in the center of his chest. It was worst if the food was hot or if he drank alcohol with his meal or after it. Hot tea, a neat whisky, or even a glass of white wine brought it on. At the same time, his heartburn was more severe than before and lasted longer. He was going through more white bottles every week and was also taking anti-indigestion tablets by the dozen.

This deterioration was gradual, so even the new intensity of pain did not cause him to seek his doctor's advice. He had to be shocked into doing that. When he got out of bed one morning, he felt dizzy and faint. He staggered to the toilet, where he passed a stool the color and consistency of warm tar. He looked pale and felt cold and clammy. He knew this could not be right, so he called the emergency number.

It was lucky that he did, because the black stool was a sign of bleeding. The bleeding had come from an ulcer in his esophagus. Over the years, his esophagus had become chronically inflamed from the backflow, or reflux, of acid from his stomach, and the inflammation had eventually eroded into a blood vessel. James had been on the edge of a precipice for many months and now was in immediate danger of dying from a massive internal hemorrhage.

His story has a happy ending. James was rushed to the hospital, where intensive medical treatment saved his life. He is now under constant medical supervision and is being persuaded to change his lifestyle—mainly his eating and drinking habits—by a new partner, who is a much better cook than James is!

James's hernia was complicated by the fact that he also suf-fered from *Barrett's esophagus* (also called Barrett's syndrome), a condition in which the lowest region of the esophagus is much more prone than normal to ulceration (explained in more detail in chapter 3). Suffice it to say that the combination of Barrett's esophagus and hiatus hernia can at times be life threatening. Besides causing bleeding, the combined conditions can also perfo-rate, enabling the stomach contents to be expelled into the chest cavity, where they cause a very severe, acute illness. James could have paid for his relative self-neglect with his life.

Jane's Story

Bleeding caused by *esophagitis* (inflammation of the esophagus) need not be as dramatic as in James's case, but it can, in the long term, be just as severe. Jane, at sixty-two, had known she had a hiatus hernia for years, but she was happy that she had it under good control. About five years before, she'd had what she called "a flare-up," with the typical heartburn, waterbrash, and swallowing problems described in Mary's case. However, it had settled down with medical treatment, and she had gradually drifted away from her doctor's care, deciding to buy her antacids and ranitidine over the counter and to do her own thing, rather than spend time wait-ing in line for prescriptions. She was a busy woman, and with a small florist's shop to manage she had other things to do with her time.

She still suffered the odd bout of heartburn but tended to ignore it—until just before Christmas last year, when she had a tenfold increase in her workload. Being the best and most reliable florist in her small town, she was in great demand for Christmas floral decorations and wreaths. And being a very conscientious (some might say obsessive) woman, she did all the work herself. Last year, for the first time ever, she couldn't fulfil her orders. She had to hire another woman to complete them because she was just too exhausted to carry on. After standing for an hour or so, she was dizzy, faint, and gasping for breath. She looked pale and drawn and could feel her heart racing and thumping.

Accepting at last that there was something seriously wrong, she dragged herself to her doctor. He took one look at her and tested her *hemoglobin* level—a measurement of her red blood cells. It was less than half of what it should have been.

Jane's case is quite common. Sometimes self-treatment serves only to mask the symptoms, leaving the lower end of the esophagus still irritated by the stomach's digestive juices (as explained in chapter 3). That can lead to the loss of tiny amounts of blood, every day, into the digestive system. The blood loss may be so small that it does not show obviously in the stool, but over the years it adds up. It becomes impossible for the bone marrow, which makes new red blood cells, to keep up with the extra demand, and the person becomes very anemic. Anemia may not show itself in symptoms—until there is a need to step up a gear physically. Then the need for extra oxygen can't be met unless the remaining red blood cells are asked to do at least double their usual work—which means pumping them twice as fast through the body. This forces the heart to work much harder than normal. This can be the last straw, and the result is exhaustion.

So the ramifications of a hiatus hernia extend much further than just the symptoms arising from an irritation at the lower end of the esophagus. That is why, if you have a hiatus hernia, your doctor will once in a while check on your hemoglobin level to see if you are becoming anemic. It is simply a matter of taking a small blood sample, either from a fingertip or a vein, once every three months or so.

Billy's Story

Occasionally a hiatus hernia arises in people in whom you least expect it. Billy, age twenty-five, was a fitness fanatic. He trained at his local gym five days a week. He ran, had a special routine on all the machines, and finished by lifting weights. He knew enough not to get muscle-bound and to take two days off per week to let his muscles relax and build up the stores of energy that had been used by the exercise.

So Billy was a super-fit man in peak condition. Yet he appeared in his doctor's consulting room complaining of a pain behind his breastbone and of acid regurgitation into his mouth when he bent over or lifted weights. He also found he couldn't breathe as deeply as he used to and was even getting breathless with exercise, an unheard-of problem for him. He'd had these symptoms for about a month, and they were not getting better.

It was only with more detailed questioning that he admitted that the symptoms followed a particular incident in the gym, about which he had been a bit embarrassed. He had been fooling about with friends, he said. They were comparing the strength of their stomach muscles—which in his case were pretty impressive! The challenge was to take a blow to the stomach with a medicine ball, thrown as hard as possible at close range. The first few shots were no bother to him, because he was ready for them and kept his muscles tense. But a friend had caught him unawares, with his stomach wall relaxed, and the ball had hit him squarely in the upper abdomen.

It had hurt a lot, but his macho pride kept him from admitting it, and he had rested for the next two or three days to let the pain subside. The hiatus hernia symptoms had started a few days later. This is a familiar story: a sharp blow in the abdomen with a blunt object may leave no external scars or bruises, but can rupture organs inside. Harry Houdini, the great escapologist, used to challenge people to punch him in the stomach as hard as they liked: he was always able to receive the punch with equanimity because he tensed his muscles beforehand. The one time someone punched him unexpectedly, he died from a ruptured appendix.

The same might have happened to Billy. Instead, he sustained a small rupture in his diaphragm, around the opening through which the esophagus ran. A plain X-ray (no barium was needed) showed that quite a lot of his stomach had slipped through the ruptured opening into his chest, resulting in a hiatus hernia. He needed surgery to put the stomach back into the abdomen and to repair the hole in his diaphragm. He was lucky: if his bowel had given way instead, he would have been desperately ill.

Billy's was an unusual way to bring about a hiatus hernia, but it is by no means an isolated case. Many people suffer the effects of being hit in the stomach with blunt instruments; it happens in road accidents, in falls at work, in the home, and at play. People have sustained ruptured diaphragms falling off horses, off mountains, or off ladders while doing repairs around the house or pruning fruit trees. Often they sustain other, more obvious injuries, which occupy the medical team's time, and the possibility of a diaphragm tear is missed. So if your symptoms of hiatus hernia have arisen out of the blue, try to think of any possible incident that might have caused it. Your recollection may turn out to be a pointer for your doctor to follow in his or her study of your case.

This book would not be complete without mention of two special categories of hiatus hernia—in pregnancy and in babies. The following two case histories describe them.

Liz's Story

Liz, at twenty-three, was sailing blissfully through a very successful and happy first pregnancy when she ran up against her first symptoms of hiatus hernia. It started in the sixth month, with heartburn and acid regurgitation into the mouth, especially when she was lying down. She also found she could only take small amounts of food at a time without feeling full. At night, the heartburn kept her from settling down, and even when she did drop off to sleep, she was soon wakened by it.

The cause of her symptoms was that the baby was filling her abdomen and pushing her stomach up into her chest. This didn't help her breathing either, so she became very easily breathless.

Happily, there was good news for her on two counts. First, pregnancy hiatus hernia is usually reversed as soon as the baby is born. In fact, it eases a lot in the last month, when the baby's head settles into the pelvis and leaves a little more room for the stomach to return to its normal anatomical position. Second, the hiatus hernia is relatively easily treated even during pregnancy. Remaining upright (even sleeping upright) is a great help, and several over-the-counter and prescription medicines are available that ease heartburn very quickly and reliably. Liz was given the appropriate advice and medicines, and her heartburn vanished, as promised, after the birth. She has not had it since. She was reassured that the pregnancy did no permanent damage to her diaphragm, esophagus, or stomach.

Peter's Story

Peter is three years old now, and he is a very lively and lovable little terror. It is difficult to reconcile this with the fact that he spent most of his first year strapped into a special chair to keep him upright, day and night. It took courage and patience in large measure from both parents to help him through that year.

Peter's mother first became concerned when, at about six weeks old, he started to vomit after being laid down to rest in his crib. It happened so often that she began to worry that he had some form of obstruction in the bowel. This fear was reinforced by her finding that he was no longer putting on the expected weight for a healthy baby. She spoke about her fears to a nurse, who arranged a "test feed" with the doctor.

One possible diagnosis for a six-week-old baby boy who is vomiting is *pyloric stenosis*—a benign overgrowth of muscle tissue around the outlet of the stomach into the *duodenum* (the first segment of the small intestine, immediately after the stomach). The overgrowth of muscle tissue blocks the flow of blood from the stomach to the rest of the bowel. During a test feed, the doctor can feel the overgrowth—it feels like a hazelnut—in the upper abdomen. A child with pyloric stenosis shoots vomit out like a bullet from a gun (called *projectile vomiting*), regardless of the child's posture.

However, Peter's story did not sound right for pyloric stenosis. His vomit just flowed out of his mouth, but only when he was horizontal. In Peter's case the presence of a hiatus hernia was suggested by small flecks of blood in the vomit, showing that there was already some degree of esophageal irritation from the stomach contents (described further in chapter 3).

A barium X-ray (which can be safely done on a six-week-old baby) confirmed the hernia. The next decision was what to do about it. Most early hernias like this will settle on their own if left to do so—and the way to do so was to keep Peter upright for the rest of the first year of his life! That may seem cruel, but he took to the regime beautifully. He stopped vomiting, put on plenty of weight, and developed into a healthy, normal child. Now, at three years old, he is a very lively toddler.

It is important to diagnose a congenital hiatus hernia like this early, because if it is missed or left for many months, the lower end of the esophagus can become scarred and may leave the child with a short esophagus. This leaves the junction between the esophagus and the stomach higher up than it should be—in the chest cavity rather than below the diaphragm—which may require extensive surgery later.

These aren't the only symptoms of a hiatus hernia in children. It may show itself for the first time in an older child—around a year old—as peculiar writhing movements of the neck. The parent often interprets these as some sort of fit, which naturally causes great concern and anxiety. It is only when the contortions are related to swallowing that the reason for them becomes clear. The child is using these movements in an attempt to get the food that is sticking in the esophagus down into the stomach. Children are quite conscious of what they are doing, but they are obviously not old enough to explain why.

Once the diagnosis of hiatus hernia has been made in a child and the treatment has been successful, it remains important to follow up its progress for many years—at least into adulthood. About half of all children who are treated for hiatus hernia later suffer from adult-type hiatus hernia, which must be treated properly.

The variety presented in these cases highlights the fact that hiatus hernia is not just a single condition. It has many forms, and it produces different sets of symptoms in different people. To understand why this is true, you need to know something about the normal esophagus, diaphragm, and stomach and about how the normal anatomy and architecture can go wrong. This information is provided in the next chapter.

Chapter 2

The Normal Esophagus, Diaphragm, and Stomach

The Swallowing Mechanism

In learning about the normal workings of the esophagus, the diaphragm, and the stomach, the first thing to understand is the action of normal swallowing. The only part of swallowing of which we are normally conscious happens at the back of the tongue and in the throat. From then on, after the food or drink reaches the top of the esophagus, the process is an active but unconscious one that takes place in the esophagus. It is completed when the food enters the stomach.

It is easy to imagine that the esophagus is an inactive tube through which the material we have swallowed passes, by gravity, to the stomach. However, what really happens in swallowing is very different. We transfer food towards the back of the throat (the *pharynx*) using the tongue. Once the food reaches the pharynx, swallowing becomes automatic; that is, we can feel the food in our throat, but we cannot stop the action of swallowing. The movement is now under the control of the *autonomic nervous system*, which also controls the movements of food through the rest of the gut, without our being aware of it.

We can divide the autonomic (also called *subconscious* or *involuntary*) phase of swallowing into two subphases: what goes on in the pharynx and what goes on in the esophagus.

In the Pharynx

When food or drink hits the pharynx (the back of the throat), it stimulates two muscle reflexes: one shuts off the passages back into the mouth, the back of the nose, and the lungs; the other squeezes the food down into the top of the esophagus. The aim of this is to ensure that we do not inhale and swallow at the same time—food in the lungs is a disaster that can lead to very sudden death.

In the Esophagus

The esophagus is a very muscular tube: the action of the autonomic nerves causes it to contract and relax in a very coordinated fashion, so that it actively pushes solids and liquids onwards into the stomach. These rippling muscle contractions, called *peristalsis*, occur through the whole length of the gut, from esophagus to anus, and are the means by which food, and then feces, are passed onwards. If that process fails, the food just sticks. Any liquid may trickle downwards, but solids will stay in a lump, stretching the tube walls and causing considerable discomfort.

There are three recognizable types of muscle contraction in the esophagus.

1. Once we start to swallow, primary peristaltic waves ripple down the esophagus, pushing food in front of them at a rate of five centimeters per second.

2. If the primary peristaltic waves don't manage to empty the contents of the esophagus into the stomach, then a secondary peristaltic wave starts, about halfway down the esophagus. This reinforces the primary wave, and sometimes it can be felt as an uncomfortable, almost

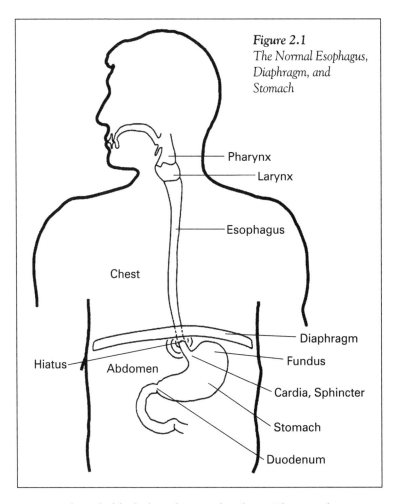

Figure 2.1
The Normal Esophagus, Diaphragm, and Stomach

Pharynx

Larynx

Esophagus

Chest

Diaphragm

Fundus

Hiatus

Abdomen

Cardia, Sphincter

Stomach

Duodenum

indescribable feeling deep in the chest. This may have been, for example, the reason for the discomfort in Eve's case (see chapter 1).

3. Tertiary muscle contractions in the esophagus have been identified by radiologists, who have vast experience of watching barium-swallow X-rays. These occur in one segment of the esophagus at a time; they don't appear to be involved in swallowing, and they don't propel food onwards. Their purpose is unknown; it is

possible that they are simply a way of keeping the muscles in tone between meals while waiting for the next lump of food to come down.

Peristalsis—both primary and secondary—is vital for transferring solid and semisolid food from the back of the pharynx into the stomach. As long as we are upright when we drink, however, peristalsis isn't absolutely necessary for liquids. Once we have swallowed a liquid, as long as there is no obstruction to its flow, it will reach the stomach by gravity alone. However, peristalsis is needed to ensure that food does not return to the throat. Without peristalsis, if you were to swallow while lying flat or standing on your head, the food or drink would flow back into your mouth.

I have very graphic memories of being taught at medical school about the way the esophagus works. Our physiology lecturer, Dr. Hilary Harries, brought into the lecture hall a pint of beer, climbed onto the demonstration table, stood on his head, facing us, then drank the beer in one go, upside down. He had no difficulty doing so, and he did not spill a drop! He declined to perform an encore.

So the rippling muscles in the wall of the esophagus ensure that passage of food and drink is one-way only. This is very important: if food travels in the opposite direction, not only do you throw it up, but you feel terrible.

At its lower end, the esophagus passes through a hole—the *hiatus*—in the *diaphragm*, which is the sheet of muscle that separates the contents of the chest from those of the abdomen (the diaphragm is described more fully later in the chapter). Below the diaphragmatic hiatus, the esophagus becomes the upper part of the stomach. How it does so, and how it relates to the diaphragm, are crucial in determining whether or not a patient has a hiatus hernia.

The Junction of Esophagus and Stomach

If it is important that food flows in a one-way direction within the esophagus, it is even more vital that, once it has reached the stomach, it stays there, and can only travel onwards into the duodenum. The digestive juices inside the stomach are very acidic and are designed to digest proteins. The stomach wall is extremely well protected against its own juices with a thick layer of mucus (to protect against the protein-digesting enzymes) and bicarbonate (to protect against the acid). However, the esophagus is not at all protected in this way; gastric juices that get into the esophagus are a powerful irritant. They can cause ulcers, inflammation, friability, and eventual scarring at the lower end of the esophagus (as discussed in chapter 3).

Therefore, several mutually cooperative mechanisms exist which act to ensure that once food has entered the stomach, it can't flow backwards, up into the esophagus.

The Cardia

The lower five centimeters or so of the esophagus lie under the diaphragm within the abdominal cavity (see Figure 2.1). The esophagus meets the stomach at its upper right-hand surface, not quite at the top. If the stomach were the face of a clock, and you were looking at it from the front, then the junction between the esophagus and the stomach would lie at about eleven o'clock.

This junction is called the *cardia*. It meets the stomach at an angle so that the food slides easily into the bottom 90 percent of the stomach. This process is not unlike tipping a glass when you pour your drink into it, to avoid turbulence and froth. The angle should also ensure that, if there is any reverse movement of food upward within the stomach, it passes by the entry from the esophagus and ends up in the top part of the stomach—to continue the analogy with a clock face, at the twelve o'clock area. This is called the *fundus*.

The fundus, being the uppermost part of the stomach, which is virtually like an unexpanded balloon, acts as a safety valve that gathers any gas that has been swallowed or produced in the process of digestion. It sits neatly under the diaphragm.

The Sphincter

At the cardia, just where the esophagus becomes the stomach, lies a ring of muscle, within the organ's wall. Imagine it as an elastic band around the tube, gripping it slightly and narrowing it. This is called the *gastroesophageal sphincter*. There are sphincters at several crucial sites in the gut: besides the one between esophagus and stomach, they also occur at the outlet of the stomach into the duodenum, between the small bowel and large bowel, and at the anus. They control the passage of food and food residues from one segment of the digestive tract to the next, and they prevent backflow.

So not only is the angle at which the esophagus meets the stomach important, so is the efficiency of the gastroesophageal sphincter. It opens (the ring of muscle relaxes) to let food and drink pass from esophagus to stomach, and it closes (the ring of muscle contracts) to prevent the digesting food from flowing back from stomach to esophagus. In effect, it is a one-way valve.

In addition to the sphincter muscles, another system of muscles keeps this valve structure intact. These are the *oblique-muscle fibers* in the wall of the esophagus and stomach around the sphincter, which keep esophagus and stomach at the appropriate angle to each other, in a sling-like support. Without the oblique muscles, the angle between esophagus and stomach would flatten out, and the bottom end of the esophagus would be more open to backflow pressures.

Such backflow pressures are normal when the stomach, full of food, starts its job of digestion. Like the esophagus, the stomach wall is subject to peristalsis, and although the movement is usually from the above going down, there are also chaotic churning waves, designed to mix the stomach contents thoroughly with the digestive juices. If the sphincter and the oblique-muscle fibers are not working properly, then this motion may push the stomach contents into the lower end of the esophagus—with the irritant consequences described above.

Abdominal Pressure

An essential force to prevent backflow is the positive pressure in the abdominal cavity. The biggest difference between the chest and abdominal cavities is the pressure within them: inside the chest, the pressure must be kept relatively low, or the lungs could not expand; inside the abdomen, the pressure is much higher, because external pressure on the gut helps to push its contents onward and eventually, of course, out. The organ that maintains this big differential in pressure between the abdominal and chest cavities is the diaphragm.

The Diaphragm

The diaphragm is a tough sheet of muscle that is attached in an umbrella-shaped circle around the lower margin of the ribs. Above it lie the lungs and the heart; below it lie the kidneys (on the left and right sides), the liver (on the right side), the spleen (on the left side), and all of the gut from the stomach, through the small and large bowel, to the rectum and anus. The high pressure that exists within the abdomen means that if the muscles of the diaphragm aren't working properly (either because of an inherited fault, or because they have given way under pressure), some part of the contents of the abdomen can be pushed into the chest cavity. This is what is meant by a *hernia*.

Obviously, the diaphragm is not a solid sheet of muscle; there are holes in it through which the esophagus and the main blood vessels from and to the heart (the *aorta* and *inferior vena cava*) must pass. The blood vessels lie at the back of the abdomen, just in front of the spine, but the esophagus enters nearer the front of the diaphragm, through an opening of its own—the hiatus.

To make sure that nothing can slip upward from the abdomen into the chest cavity through the hiatus—that is, between the outside wall of the esophagus and the surrounding circular rim of the hiatus—there are powerful muscles in the hiatus's rim that hold it close to the esophagus. These are the *diaphragmatic crura* (plural *crurae*)—a word that comes from the Latin for *cross*—so-called because they crisscross around the esophagus, keeping it tightly and effectively in place. Under normal circumstances, nothing can pass between the crural edges and the outer esophageal surface.

This is a very useful setup, not only for preventing a hernia, but also for ensuring that the external pressure around the lower few centimeters of the esophagus (the part that lies inside the abdomen) remains high. So, even if the cardia is slightly inefficient and could possibly let stomach contents pass back into the esophagus, this is prevented purely by the high external pressure, which effectively keeps the esophagus collapsed until the pressure of food and peristalsis from above opens it up. In fact, this positive pressure exerted on the lower end of the esophagus is probably the most important mechanism for preventing the backflow of stomach contents into it. When the cardia is pushed up into the chest cavity—as happens with a hernia—where the pressure surrounding it is much lower, then backflow from stomach to esophagus becomes the rule, rather than the exception.

If you have read this far without having to reread some sections, congratulations! You will have realized by now that what goes on in the act of swallowing and what occurs where the esophagus meets the stomach are complex. A summary of the processes described in this chapter may be useful.

In brief: the esophagus, in a series of muscular movements, pushes the food down through the diaphragm, where the crura ensures that no unwanted return of food occurs. Just below the diaphragm, the pressure on the last portion of esophagus reinforces that function, so the food passes into the stomach through the cardia. There, the angle between the lower end of the esophagus and the stomach, along with the sphincter and the oblique muscles around the opening to the stomach, all combine to ensure that the food enters the stomach and cannot return. It is a perfect system—if it works! If it doesn't, there is trouble. This is explained in chapter 3.

Chapter 3

Hiatus Hernia and Related Problems

lthough this book is mainly about hiatus hernias, it also covers conditions that are not strictly a form of hiatus hernia but which for convenience are labeled as such. Many people, for example, have a hernia in another part of the diaphragm, usually next to the hiatus: strictly speaking, this is a *paraesophageal hernia* or *rolling hernia*, but it is usually called *hiatus hernia* for simplicity. There are subtle differences between the symptoms of hiatus hernia and those of paraesophageal hernia. These were described in the case histories of chapter 1 and are explained in this chapter.

However, there are also conditions involving the esophagus that mimic hiatus hernia: the symptoms are very similar, but no hernia is actually present. For example, acid reflux can spread up from the stomach without there being an actual hernia, or "pouches" in the wall of the esophagus can fill with food or gas and mimic a rolling hernia. These, too, are described in this chapter, since many people who have what they think is hiatus hernia may actually be suffering from one of them.

To fully understand the differences between these conditions, you need to know a little about how the esophagus develops in the embryo and where the process can go wrong.

The Beginnings: How Trouble Can Develop

The esophagus is first recognizable in the thirty-five-day-old embryo as a one-millimeter-long, vertical, solid cylinder with a groove along each side. As it grows, the groove splits the cylinder into two tubes, the front half becoming the breathing tubes—the trachea and main bronchus—and the back half becoming the swallowing apparatus—the esophagus. By the time the baby is born, these two tubes are hollow and completely separate from one another, so that the baby can breathe and swallow without the one system interfering with the other.

Occasionally, the separation is incomplete. This can lead to several conditions:

* to open tubes that join the esophagus to the breathing system—these are called *tracheoesophageal fistulae*;

* to a blind end on the esophagus so that it does not meet up with the stomach at all (called *tracheoesophageal atresia*);

* to a congenital esophageal hernia, in which the cardia (explained in chapter 2 as the junction between the esophagus and the stomach) lies above the diaphragm, along with a portion of stomach. This is, in fact, an unusual form of hiatus hernia.

Surgery for Newborn Babies

These conditions are usually very obvious in the first few days of life, as the baby has difficulty feeding. The main problem is vomiting or regurgitation of food. Children with tracheoesophageal fistulae go blue and choke during their first feeding as food spills into their lungs—so diagnosis is usually made very quickly. Surgery must be performed to close off the connection between the two tubes before these babies are fed again.

Surgery soon after birth may also be necessary if a baby has a large hiatus hernia. This condition can sometimes mean that a large portion of the organs that should be in the abdominal cavity are instead inside the chest. This can make a baby very breathless and distressed, especially when lying down. Sitting the baby up, so that gravity causes the organs to return to the abdomen, can cause an instant improvement. However, emergency surgery is needed to return the abdominal organs to their proper positions and to close off the hole in the diaphragm.

During the operation, whether it is for a fistula or a hiatus hernia, the surgeon ensures that the esophagus is long enough to reach the stomach below the diaphragm, that the diaphragm is intact, and that the cardia, below the diaphragm, is working correctly. This is essential even in the case of a tracheoesophageal fistula, because many such children have future trouble with a hiatus hernia. It is best if it can be prevented by the correct surgery at birth.

The Early Start—and the Later Problems

Being born with a tracheoesophageal fistula is much less common than being born with a hiatus hernia. Dr. B. T. Johnston and his colleagues reported in 1995 on the follow-up of 192 children brought to the Royal Belfast Hospital for Sick Children between 1945 and 1972 for treatment of hiatus hernia. All the children had been admitted because of vomiting and regurgitation of food. Of those who were treated medically, as opposed to undergoing surgery, two-thirds had started medical treatment (in the form of the postural-chair system mentioned in Peter's story in chapter 1) before the age of six months; the rest were treated when they were between six and eighteen months old.

Of the 118 cases who could be traced, 94 had not undergone surgery in childhood, and 24 had. How did they manage as adults? Of those who had not had surgery, more than half of those who agreed to undergo a barium X-ray (76 adults) still had a hiatus hernia; 43 of the 94 still had heartburn at least once a month. However, their symptoms depended to some extent on how they had responded to their medical treatment as children. Only 20 percent of those who had responded well to postural treatment as babies still needed regular antacid treatment as adults—in contrast to 46 percent of those who had not fared so well as children. However, even members of this latter group were managing fairly well: only three of them found that their heartburn was interfering with their daily activities.

Of the 24 adults in the follow-up who had needed surgery in childhood for their hiatus hernias, 14 had been over four years old when they were first seen by the hospital; by this time they already had scarring of their lower esophagus. This suggests a strong need to give children proper treatment as early in life as possible. Eighteen of the 24 adults were still experiencing heartburn at least once a month, and 13 at least once a week. Of the 20 who agreed to a barium X-ray, 17 still had a hiatus hernia.

A crucial point made by the authors of this study was that early recognition and treatment of hiatus hernia is very important for long-term success. Of the children treated before they were six months old, 72 percent had what was assessed as a very good outcome—as compared to 29 percent of those whose treatment started after age six months.

What about the figures for heartburn in these adults who'd had hiatus hernias as children? Superficially they look bad, with about half of them suffering regular heartburn. In fact, these numbers are no worse than those for the general population. In five large European and North American population surveys, reported from 1976 to 1991, the proportion of "normal" people who had heartburn (not necessarily treated by antacids) at least once a month ranged from a minimum of 20 percent to a maximum of 44 percent. In the Belfast group, 33 percent were still taking antacids for heartburn at least once a month. The corresponding figures for the rest of the community, according to the surveys, ranged from 27 percent to 32 percent.

What did the authors conclude from their study? The main conclusion was that children with hiatus hernias should be treated as early as possible, using the postural method to begin with. If that is not successful, surgery is a second resort—but the decision to operate should be made early, rather than later, when the esophagus might already be scarred by constant exposure to acid.

They also concluded that children who respond to treatment do very well as adults, in that their quality of life is no different from that of the rest of the population, even if they still have a hiatus hernia. This, of course, raises the question of how many of the general population actually have a hiatus hernia without knowing it? How many of the 40 percent or so of us who suffer regularly from heartburn actually have a hiatus hernia?

The answer is probably academic. After all, it is the symptoms caused by the hiatus hernia, rather than the hernia itself, that matter to people. If we can get rid of the symptoms, the existence of even a small hernia does not matter. The medical argument about the proportion of the population with a hiatus hernia has been going on since 1925, when Dr. L. B. Morrison, an American radiologist, reported that 1 percent of all adults surveyed had a hiatus hernia, according to his X-ray findings. This falls far short of the number who have heartburn—the major symptom of a hiatus hernia—but many instances must occur of small hernias that failed to show up on Dr. Morrison's system of tests.

The same is likely true for childhood. Medical experts are beginning to believe that many people have had hiatus hernias from a very early age and that most hernias do not cause symptoms until adulthood. Most people respond well to the proper medical treatment, avoiding the need for surgery. A description of the symptoms and a discussion about deciding between surgery and medical treatment alone are offered later in the book.

Barrett's Esophagus

One condition must be mentioned before we progress to a wider discussion of what goes wrong in hiatus hernia and that is Barrett's esophagus. In 1950, British surgeon N. R. Barrett wrote a paper titled "Chronic Peptic Ulcer of the Oesophagus and Oesophagitis." It was published in the *British Journal of Surgery*—and since then, the name Barrett's esophagus (or Barrett's syndrome) has always been given to such cases.

People with Barrett's esophagus experience two main symptoms: they have heartburn (usually severe), and their food tends to "come back" into the throat (regurgitation). Even when they have not eaten recently, they find bitter gastric secretions welling up into their mouth. If the condition continues without treatment, they develop difficulties in swallowing (*dysphagia*), and they also start to experience a severe, boring pain in the center of the chest, which can travel through to the back. The first is a sign that scarring in the esophagus is causing an area of narrowing (a stricture) beyond which food cannot pass easily. The second is a sign of a peptic ulcer in the esophagus. Both are very serious signs. People in this state *must* be treated, as the next stage can be bleeding (hemorrhage) from the ulcer or even perforation of the ulcer into the chest cavity, with all the damage that can be wrought if the lungs are exposed to the stomach's digestive juices.

In Barrett's esophagus, the flaw is in the lining of the lower end of the esophagus. Instead of the usual tough, skinlike cells that line the normal esophagus, the lining is much more like the lining of the stomach wall, with glands and other cells that are much more susceptible to acid attack but which do not produce adequate amounts of protective mucus. Since the Barrett's esophagus is often also associated with a hiatus hernia, it is repeatedly exposed to stomach acid and pepsin. The ensuing irritation and inflammation lead to the strictures and ulcers. There are even acid-producing cells in the Barrett's tissue itself—so it contains the mechanism of its own destruction.

Obviously, people with Barrett's esophagus are at more danger than others with an uncomplicated hiatus hernia—and without tests it is difficult to tell, just from the symptoms, one from the other, particularly in the early stages. This is one reason why most people with relatively severe hiatus hernia symptoms are asked to undergo a series of quite unpleasant tests, to make sure of the diagnosis. The tests are described in chapter 6.

Why people have a Barrett's esophagus in the first place is still a matter of argument among experts. It was initially thought to be a congenital defect—people were born with the wrong type of lining in the lower esophagus—but opinion has swung to the belief that it may be an acquired condition after birth, although what causes it to be acquired is unknown.

Twenty-two years of studying patients with symptoms of hiatus hernia led American surgeons J. Borrie and L. Goldwater to report that 4.5 percent of these patients have a Barrett's esophagus. Oddly, they fall into two main age groups: children from birth to fifteen years old and adults from forty-eight to eighty years old. Three times as many men as women have a Barrett's esophagus, and there are several reports of families in which more than one member has it.

Barrett's esophagus has been linked with cancer, but this too is a source of argument among the experts. There have been repeated, but isolated, reports of people who have both Barrett's esophagus and esophageal cancer. The biggest series of studies is from the Mayo Clinic in the United States, where Dr. A. J. Cameron and colleagues found, among 122 patients with Barrett's esophagus, that 18 of them (almost 15 percent) also had esophageal cancer.

This sounds very conclusive, but in more than eight years of follow-up of the remaining 104 patients, only two further cancers were found. In another series, reported by S. J. Spechler and colleagues, just two patients, out of a total of 105 with Barrett's esophagus, developed esophageal cancer in a follow-up over three years. Both were heavy smokers and alcoholics who either refused to, or were unable to, stop their habits. Taking the two series together, the esophageal cancer rate was more than 40 times that expected of people without any known esophageal disease—but it remains a small risk in absolute terms.

The risk is even lower if it is considered that, of the patients with Barrett's esophagus in these studies, 85 percent were cigarette smokers and 76 percent were, in the words of the authors, "addicted to alcohol." As these two social habits are both known to raise the risks of esophageal cancer and may even be partly instrumental in causing Barrett's esophagus in the first place, it is difficult to calculate the risk, if any, of cancer in the patient with Barrett's esophagus who is a nonsmoker and drinks only a little.

What these figures do mean is that if you are a smoker and a heavy drinker, the first thing you must do is to stop both of those habits. My hints for quitting smoking are set forth in chapter 7.

Types of Hiatus Hernia

In medicine, as in many sciences, the pendulum of expert opinion swings to and fro as facts become clear and cherished theories are disproved. Fifty years ago, most experts held that most people with heartburn had a hiatus hernia. If the usual methods of identifying one did not show it, then it was assumed that the methods were too crude to do so, but it was accepted that one was probably present, nevertheless.

As techniques for X-ray and for endoscopic examination (passing a flexible fiber-optic tube into the stomach; explained in chapter 6) became more sophisticated and things inside the body could be seen in more detail, that opinion was gradually replaced by a view that acid could flow back (*reflux*) into the esophagus without a hernia present. The theory held that at times the esophageal sphincter relaxed, allowing reflux. Evidence also existed, from a series of cases reported in 1968, that there were many people with hiatus hernias who had never had symptoms.

However, new evidence suggests that the relaxation of the sphincter is not as important as was previously believed and that most heartburn is indeed caused by a hernia. The problem lies in identifying a small hernia—it is certainly not true that the bigger the hernia the worse it is. In fact, in many cases the reverse is the

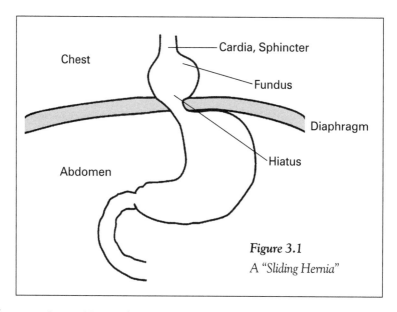

Figure 3.1
A *"Sliding Hernia"*

case. In a 1981 study, researchers showed by using special X-ray techniques that 90 percent of people with esophagitis (inflammation of the esophagus) did indeed have a hiatus hernia, but that in many cases it was a small one.

The Sliding Hernia

Figure 3.1 shows what happens with a sliding hernia (see chapter 2 for an explanation of the different body parts and of a properly working system). The basic fault is that the junction between the esophagus and the stomach (the cardia) does not lie below the diaphragm, in the abdominal cavity, but in the chest. This means that all of the mechanisms preventing the reflux of stomach contents into the esophagus are lost. The esophagus now enters the stomach at its uppermost point—at twelve o'clock instead of eleven o'clock—so that no fundal compartment exists in the stomach to collect gas and to keep the pressures in the stomach low. Instead, the esophagus enters straight into the top of the stomach, with a round opening, instead of the normal angled oval, so there is no "flap" valve to prevent reflux. There is no diaphragmatic crura to close off the lower end of the esophagus and no sling mechanism to support the junction between esophagus and stomach. Some of the stomach is in the chest, so there are cells in the chest directly producing digestive juices, allowing free access to the esophageal cells above.

It took a study using both X-rays and pressure measurements inside the esophagus to clarify what happens during swallowing in people with a sliding hiatus hernia. F. H. Longi and P. H. Jordan showed that if people with a sliding hiatus hernia were asked to swallow some barium and then to swallow a second time, barium that had collected in the hernia flowed back into the esophagus as the sphincter opened to receive the second swallow.

Longi and Jordan proposed that this meant that a small amount of acid is trapped in a hernia at one swallow and then is ejected up into the esophagus with the next. This type of reverse movement is not present in people who have no hiatus hernia or in people with a very large hernia.

This study (and others since that have confirmed its findings) helps to rectify what appears at first illogical—that small hiatus hernias are more likely to cause symptoms than large ones. One reason for this is that according to a law of physics (Laplace's law), the pressure inside a sphere is inversely proportional to its radius; in other words, the larger the hernia, the lower is the pressure inside it. And the lower the pressure, the less is the force pushing its contents upward. If the diameter of the hernia is much greater than that of the esophagus (the hernia can "balloon" in size), no reflux can occur from hernia to esophagus.

Also, small hernias are more likely to have a smaller opening and to retain the pressure inside them for longer, so they retain their contents for longer, and the potential for irritation is much greater. The pressure inside them is likely to be higher, so if the sphincter is not working, or is relaxed, then backflow is more likely to occur into the esophagus. Such small hernias may well have been missed by past types of investigation. They are less likely to be missed today.

How they are investigated is explained in chapter 6, although it has to be said here that only a minority of people with hiatus hernia symptoms need such extra tests. When approaching your doctor for the first time with symptoms, you must expect her or him to make a diagnosis and to start you on a regimen of medical treatment and lifestyle changes before considering embarking upon intrusive investigations. You will only need these if you do not respond well to the initial therapy, and nowadays that is, thankfully, fairly rare.

The Rolling Hernia

About 5 percent of all hiatus hernias are "rollers" (or parae-sophageal hernias) rather than "sliders." In these cases, the fundus of the stomach "rolls" up into the chest to lie alongside the lower end of the esophagus (see Figure 3.2). The cardia remains below the diaphragm and still works well. The angle between lower esophagus and stomach remains in place—as do all the other mechanisms, such as the sphincter and the diaphragmatic crura—so reflux of stomach contents into the esophagus does not take place.

The description may sound as if a rolling hernia is not as bad as a sliding hernia, since it does not cause heartburn or regurgitation, but that is not necessarily the case, because other symptoms can be worse. With a rolling hernia, quite a large portion of the stomach can be displaced into the chest, and there may even be loops of intestine in the sac that can fill with gas.

In this case (in contrast to a sliding hernia), the larger the hernia, the worse the symptoms. The distension of the part of the stomach that enters the chest can cause considerable pain and a very uncomfortable bloated feeling—and the more distended it is, the more likely it is to become obstructed at the site of the opening in the diaphragm. The only way to relieve the pain and distension is by belching and vomiting; this is what wakes people in the night to roam around the house until the symptoms can be relieved.

Even worse, a paraesophageal hernia can be so large that it

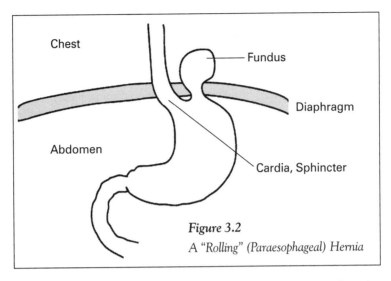

Chest

Fundus

Diaphragm

Abdomen

Cardia, Sphincter

Figure 3.2
A "Rolling" (Paraesophageal) Hernia

takes up space normally used by the heart and lungs, so that the sufferer becomes extremely breathless (feeling unable to draw a deep enough breath) and the heart begins to beat erratically. Only surgery can help at this stage.

In fact, the main treatment for all rolling hernias is surgical repair of the hole in the diaphragm through which the hernia has occurred. Even if the hole is relatively small, an early operation is advised to prevent it from growing suddenly bigger. It is far better to operate on a hernia under control than to have to operate in an emergency on a person with a blocked gut inside a chest in which both the lungs and heart are in distress!

Esophageal Spasm: Achalasia and Other Disorders

A description of the conditions that cause the symptoms of hiatus hernia would not be complete if it lacked what doctors know as "functional disorders of the esophagus." These are not hiatus hernias but are problems with the muscles of the esophagus, resulting in a disturbance of the normal process of peristalsis, which pushes the food into the stomach. With these conditions, no obvious anatomical defect exists in the esophagus, diaphragm, cardia, or stomach—but the lack of muscle coordination can create havoc with the swallowing process.

Achalasia

The most common condition is achalasia. Achalasia can start at any age, from childhood onward. The main symptom is difficulty in swallowing (dysphagia). At first, the sufferer finds it easier to swallow liquids than solids, but after a while, most food and drink seem to stick in the chest. If this state is allowed to continue, the esophagus distends and fills with food, which can suddenly reappear in the mouth. That is bad enough, but if it occurs during sleep, you can breathe the food in. If this does not choke you, it will at least cause severe irritation in the lungs. In some achalasia sufferers, the main symptom is repeated chest infections from minor bouts of food inhalation. In the early stages of achalasia, barium X-rays show only a bulging lower esophagus above a short, narrowed segment that will not open. Later, the bulge grows much bigger, and the esophagus can eventually become like a large, soft, twisted bag full of undigested food.

Achalasia is thought to be caused by the failure of the peristaltic wave to pass through the lowest segment of the esophagus, which remains narrow and underdeveloped. There seems to be a fault at this segment in the muscles of the esophageal wall, or in the nerves that control their contraction and relaxation. In the early stages of achalasia, the narrowed region can be stretched successfully by an instrument called a *bougie,* or a water-filled dilator, but most cases need surgery to refashion the cardia so that its muscles allow the passage of food from esophagus to stomach. This is called *anterior myotomy,* or the modified Heller operation.

Sadly, one occasional aftereffect of the Heller operation is the startup of reflux from stomach to esophagus, so that one set of symptoms is replaced by another. However, the relief from the first is so good that the vast majority find the second trivial in comparison.

Three other esophageal problems related to achalasia include diffuse spasm, nutcracker esophagus, and tertiary contractions.

Diffuse Spasm

With *diffuse spasm*, the peristaltic wave is normal, but from time to time an extra contraction occurs, during which the whole esophagus in effect goes into cramp. The muscles along the length of the esophagus contract and stay contracted for minutes at a time. This causes a deep-seated central-chest pain that is often mistaken for angina or even a heart attack. Treatment is described in the section on nutcracker esophagus, below.

Nutcracker Esophagus

With *nutcracker esophagus*, the peristaltic wave—normally a strictly unconscious process—is intensified to a much higher strength and a much longer duration. It is so intense that it is felt as a very severe pain, as if the cramping muscles could crack a nut inside them. X-rays taken at the time of the pain show very intense waves of contractions of the muscles in the esophageal wall.

Both diffuse spasm and nutcracker esophagus can be very difficult to treat. Antispasmodic drugs may help, but for relief of symptoms some people require regular insertion of a bougie into the esophagus or even an operation to cut the esophageal muscles. (See chapter 9 for descriptions of these procedures.)

It is thought that some of the spasms occurring in diffuse spasm and in nutcracker esophagus are initiated when small amounts of acid pass, by reflux, up from the stomach into the lower esophagus. In such patients the esophageal lining appears to be extremely sensitive to such acid, and the muscles around it respond accordingly, either with cramping or with exaggerated peristalsis that spreads through the whole length of the esophagus.

Tertiary Contractions

Tertiary contractions are a series of uncoordinated contractions of segments of esophagus; they do not aid the propulsion of food toward the stomach. They are linked in some patients with reflux, but they are also seen in older patients with no obvious symptoms. An extreme degree of tertiary spasms can result in corkscrew esophagus, in which the whole esophagus twists on itself. Although that sounds horrendous, it hardly ever causes severe symptoms and can be revealed by chance in X-rays of patients being investigated for reasons other than esophageal symptoms. Tertiary contractions rarely need any form of treatment.

Chapter 4

The Doctor's Diagnosis

Having read the first three chapters, you will by now understand that hiatus hernia is not a single diagnosis, but a group of complex conditions with different symptoms and different underlying processes that require different treatments. The case histories in chapter 1 and the potential problems with the esophagus, diaphragm, cardia, and stomach set forth in chapter 3 should have convinced you of the importance of being able to describe your symptoms to your doctor with some degree of accuracy. If you can't do that, it will take longer for your doctor to unravel the facts and match them to a diagnosis. If you wish, reread the case histories to see how much they differ from one another—and yet they all come under the diagnosis of "hiatus hernia."

Keep in mind that most general practitioners will make an initial, probable diagnosis from what their patients tell them and from a modest examination of the chest and abdomen. For most patients that is enough, and no further tests are necessary before treatment can begin. In a few patients, the presence of certain warning symptoms and signs will prompt the doctor to take things further, probably by referring the patient to a specialist gastroenterologist. Sometimes, however, the symptoms turn out to be caused by something else and not at all by a hiatus hernia or esophageal disease (this is discussed in chapter 5).

Your Doctor's Questions

Most people, when they have plucked up the courage to face their doctor with a problem, do so because of one main symptom they have found intolerable or excessively worrisome. Once you admit to this symptom, your doctor will try to link it with others, so you will be asked a series of questions designed to produce a response that will fit a particular diagnosis.

For the person with a probable hiatus hernia, the main symptom is likely to be heartburn—but as our case histories illustrate, symptoms can also range from an odd sensation of discomfort, to regurgitation of food or fluid, to difficulty in swallowing, or even to bleeding. The questions you will be asked will therefore take the following pattern.

On Heartburn

So you have heartburn? Can you describe it in more detail?

For example, is it truly a searing or burning pain, or is it more a dull ache?

Exactly where is it? Does it stay behind the breastbone, or does it move up into the jaw or into the arm (particularly the left arm)? Does it appear in the pit of the stomach or travel into the back?

Does it come on with eating? If so, does the amount of food make a difference? Or the type of food?

Your answers to these questions will already have narrowed down the options. The quality of the pain matters a lot: a burning pain points to acid in the esophagus; a dull ache may mean the development of an esophageal ulcer, or even pain from the heart. The distribution of the pain matters: the more widespread it is, the more extensive the esophageal irritation, and the more likely it is that you will need more intensive treatment. Burning esophageal pain, like angina, can spread into the jaw, arm, and stomach—but if your pain is more dull and aching than burning, and extends into these areas, then your doctor will be considering angina as another diagnosis.

Heartburn-like pain with eating (particularly if it is almost immediate) is usually esophageal, and the larger the meal the more likely it is to cause symptoms. But that is also true for some types of angina, so the fact that your dull ache is brought on by food does not rule out angina. The interval between starting to eat and the onset of pain, however, is usually longer for angina and for stomach ulcer—another diagnosis likely to be in the doctor's mind. Paradoxically, hunger may also bring on heartburn; this fact does tend to differentiate it from angina (but not from a stomach ulcer). As for the types of food most likely to bring on heartburn, alcohol, spices, raw fruit, carbonated drinks, and hot drinks (especially tea without milk) top my patients' list.

On Posture

Do your symptoms get worse when you adopt any particular posture? For example, when you're stooping, bending, lying down?

Do they come on when you're lifting heavy weights?

How comfortable are you in bed? Do you have to sleep propped up?

Are you wakened at night with heartburn?

If you have a sliding hernia, your symptoms are likely to be greatly influenced by the position you adopt. If the pain starts when you stoop, bend over, or lie down, this strongly suggests hiatus hernia with reflux. The symptoms are often worst in bed, and many people have already found, long before they seek their doctor's help, that sleeping in a propped-up position eases the symptoms.

Many people tend to prop up the head of the bed with blocks, but that can lead to their sliding down the bed during sleep and waking up in the middle of the night with heartburn because they are by then lying flat. It is best to put a blocking board at the foot of the bed, so that your feet come up against it, to prevent you from sliding down any farther. Better yet, put blocks under the foot of the bed and an angled support under your pillows, so that your torso rests at an angle of around 60 degrees from horizontal and your legs are at around 10 degrees. Then, any tendency to slide while you are asleep will be towards the head of the bed, thereby reinforcing the angle and keeping you relatively upright while sleeping.

On "Discomfort" or Other Pain

Do you have pain or discomfort other than, or in addition to, the heartburn?

If so, how can you best describe it? Exactly where is it?

What brings it on?

The most common pain apart from heartburn is a discomfort often described as a raw feeling or an aching pain, or simply as a discomfort for which there are no more accurate words, felt mainly in the back of the throat or in the upper, central part of the chest just behind the breastbone. Although it is not usually as severe as heartburn, it is made worse by swallowing food or hot or cold liquids. This painful swallowing can be a sign of acute esophagitis, which may have been caused by a recent drinking bout or by overindulgence in spicy food! It does not usually last long, as acute esophagitis settles quickly—but heed it as a warning against future dietary indiscretions.

A constant ache in the center of the chest, which is not particularly made worse by food but may be worsened by hunger, may be a sign of an ulcer in an irritated esophagus and must be taken seriously.

On Regurgitation

Do you find food or drink that you have just swallowed coming back into your mouth? (This is quite different from vomiting,

*in which you first feel sick, and then the stomach muscles
contract to heave the food up from the mouth forcefully out-
ward. The regurgitation from a hiatus hernia wells up without a feeling of nausea.)*

If you do regurgitate, how soon after swallowing does it happen?

*Does it have the same taste as when it went down, or is there an
added sour or bitter taste?*

Does it come with belching and gas?

Are you bothered by regurgitation at night, when lying flat?

Do you get breathless, and are you prone to chest infections?

The answers to these questions are important, because they can
indicate how serious your problem is and whether there is a need
to operate rather than just use medical treatment. For example,
regurgitation immediately after swallowing, combined with the
lack of a sour or bitter taste, suggests that there is a blockage in the
esophagus—possibly a stricture from old scarring or from achalasia. A bitter or sour taste confirms that stomach contents are
entering the esophagus—so there is reflux. Belching is also an
indication that stomach contents are involved. Bile—an excessively bitter-tasting green liquid in the regurgitated material—
means that even the outlet of the stomach into the duodenum is
not functioning properly. In this case, further tests are mandatory,
as there may be obstruction lower down in the gut.

Regurgitation at night is also a very important indication for
further tests. If you regurgitate when you are sleeping, you may
breathe some of the contents into your lungs. Two American surveys reported respectively that 60 percent and 40 percent of
patients with hiatus hernias had serious, chronic lung disorders
such as bronchitis, asthma, *bronchiectasis* (in which there are mul-
tiple pockets of infection deep within the lung), and pneumonia.
By 1979 the connection between night regurgitation and lung disease was being questioned. In that year, C. A. Pellegrini and col-

leagues studied 48 hiatus hernia patients whom they suspected were breathing regurgitated food into their lungs: only 8 of them were actually doing so, 5 of whom had a primary lung disorder quite separate from their hernia.

The experts continue to argue about the importance of regurgitation at night. My own feeling is that if it happens to you, surgery should be strongly considered—particularly if you have any chest symptoms. I base this on the evidence of T. L. Lomasney, who found in 1977 that surgical correction of reflux (explained in chapter 9) cured or greatly improved not only the regurgitation but also the chest problems in the vast majority of patients.

On Swallowing

Do you have difficulty with swallowing?

Does it feel as if food is stuck inside your chest?

How often does this happen? Is it getting worse?

The feeling that food isn't slipping down as easily as it should is very common with hiatus hernia. It can mean one of two problems. When it "comes and goes," this is usually a sign of esophagitis—irritation of the esophagus due to acid regurgitation. When the acid is removed with medication, the condition rapidly improves. However, if it is gradually getting worse and more frequent, and especially if it happens with every meal, a stricture must be suspected and investigated. Strictures are fixed, permanent narrowings of the esophagus, which are usually the end result of many episodes of esophagitis. The repeated inflammation and healing eventually produces scars that contract and constrict the diameter of the esophagus and that do not open up, even under pressure. Such strictures may occur anyplace along the esophagus.

Some swallowing difficulties are due to spasm of segments of esophageal muscles. This happens in cases of achalasia and the other muscle disorders described in chapter 3. Spasms also give the feeling that food is held up deep inside the chest, but they are also painful—and the feeling suddenly disappears, along with the pain, as the spasm eases off. However, in more severe forms of achalasia, the symptoms are so similar to those of an organic stricture that X-rays and endoscopy are needed to differentiate between them.

On Bleeding

Have you noticed any bleeding?

Is there blood in the material you bring up?

What color are your stools? Have they ever been black?

By inducing intense inflammation, esophagitis due to acid reflux may erode into the small blood vessels just under the esophageal lining. This can cause bleeding, which you will know about if you tend to regurgitate. The blood can appear as flecks of red or rusty brown in the liquid that appears in your mouth.

However, if you don't have this symptom, the only way you can detect regular bleeding from an irritated esophagus is by looking at your stools. By the time blood has traveled from the esophagus through the gut to the rectum and anus, it is changed chemically, so that it is black, rather than red. A stool containing a lot of blood is also changed in consistency; it is like soft tar rather than normally formed. If you have noticed these changes, you must tell your doctor. Black tarry stools (called *melena*) are a reason for emergency admission to the hospital so the bleeding can be stopped. You ignore them at your peril; such hemorrhages can be fatal if allowed to continue.

Not all bleeding is so obvious. The blood loss from a chronically irritated esophagus may be only a few milliliters a day. This will not show obviously in the stools; they may appear slightly darker brown than normal, but not enough to cause concern. And their consistency will not change. However, even the loss of two milliliters of blood a day, over many months, can be enough to cause anemia as the body struggles to replace the loss.

Although you will not notice the loss in the stool, modern tests for blood in the stool will pick up such small amounts. Do not be surprised, therefore, if your doctor asks for a sample of stool to test. (It is common to ask for three specimens given on three separate days, just to make sure.) You will also be asked for a blood sample so that your hemoglobin level and perhaps your reticulocyte count can be checked. The first is a measure of how much oxygen-carrying power your red cells have—and whether you are anemic. The second is a measure of how many young red cells you have—and therefore how hard your bone marrow is working to replace any loss. The higher the reticulocyte count, the harder the marrow is working to replace lost red blood cells.

Very occasionally, hiatus hernia and esophagitis can cause no symptoms—they are "silent"—so that the first sign of trouble is a hemorrhage, which appears as blood in the mouth or as melena. If it is severe, it is usually caused by an ulcer in a Barrett's esophagus (see chapter 3). It appears that the change in the lining of the lower esophagus that makes the Barrett's esophagus more susceptible to ulceration also makes it less sensitive, or even insensitive, to pain. Patients with this problem usually need surgery to remove the ulcerated area and lifelong treatment to prevent any recurrence.

On Belching and Bloating

Do you belch a lot? Do you feel bloated? How often does it happen?

Belching and bloating are embarrassing symptoms, but they are not a sign of anything dangerous. This is a comfort to some people whose bloating is so intense that they fear their stomach may burst. It won't.

It may be difficult for readers who are badly afflicted by wind to accept this, but in most cases it is caused by subconscious, excessive swallowing of air. Everyone swallows a little air from time to time, but in big gas producers, swallowing is a constant habit every few seconds—and all that can be swallowed is some saliva and a lot of air. The air must either be belched up or passed onward into the gut, where it eventually must be passed out at the other end of the digestive system.

The answer is to try to stop swallowing air. This may be much more difficult to do than it seems, because once you know you are doing it, the habit can become even more intense. You may need training in relaxation to help yourself.

Of course, everyone has some gas in the stomach; some air swallowing is essential as a normal part of digestion. If you have a hiatus hernia, this air can gather in the fundus (trapped in the chest in a rolling hernia; see chapter 3) and cause pain and discomfort deep inside the chest. The trick is to find out how best to displace the air back into the part of the stomach that remains inside the abdomen and then be able to belch it up. People differ in the ways they find to do this: some get up and roam the house in the middle of the night, others lie on a particular side, yet others have a favorite medicine (see chapter 8 for a discussion of treatment with medicines).

In the meantime, if this is happening to you constantly, then you *must* make it known to your doctor, for you may have a rolling hernia that needs surgical, rather than medical, treatment to put it right. Rolling hernias sometimes have a habit of growing much bigger quite quickly, and that can lead to an emergency as described in chapter 3. It is far better to prevent than to experience such an occurrence!

Case Histories Revisited

Let us now return to the patients described in chapter 1, this time looking at their histories from their doctor's viewpoint.

Mary had a sliding hiatus hernia with esophagitis (hence the heartburn) and eventually esophageal ulceration (hence the central persistent pain). After a few weeks of medical management and the supervised loss of 40 pounds, she underwent surgery to repair her hernia and to make sure it did not return.

Eve had a large paraesophageal hernia that from time to time filled with food or gas. Most paraesophageal hernias are operated upon, because they can grow bigger and eventually become obstructed. She was not thrilled about surgery, however, and as the symptoms had settled fairly quickly and she'd suffered only two serious bouts of the illness separated by many years, her doctor gave her case the benefit of the doubt and managed it with drugs and lifestyle advice. He did warn her, however, that if the symptoms returned, he would strongly recommend surgery.

Harry had a moderate to large sliding hernia. He has remained almost symptom-free on medical treatment. However, his hiatus hernia is not his doctor's only worry. The fact that he has experienced both gallbladder trouble and a hiatus hernia, is a bit overweight, and (it was found at the last examination) has high blood pressure puts him among the 20 percent of hiatus hernia patients with a linked disease. His doctor knows he is at higher than average risk of a peptic ulcer and of coronary heart disease, so he will be watching Harry closely for early signs of those diseases. However, now that Harry plays golf regularly, no longer smokes or crawls around under floorboards, and is losing his excess weight, he is expected to do well.

James had a Barrett's esophagus. Happily for James, the bleeding was not profuse enough to end his life before he got to the hospital! He needed emergency surgery to stop the bleeding and then further surgery a few weeks later (after intense medical treatment to heal the esophagitis) to remove the ulcer-bearing area.

Jane's diagnosis (remember that she was anemic from constant small bleeds) was not absolutely clear-cut. She might have had a stomach or duodenal ulcer—remember that one in five hiatus hernia sufferers also has an ulcer—or the bleeding could have come, by coincidence, from elsewhere in the gut. So Jane had to undergo investigations to ensure that all the possibilities were ruled out. Happily, in her case, she settled satisfactorily on long-term medical treatment for her esophagitis. There was no need for surgery, but she promised to return to her doctor for a regular checkup, initially every three months, mainly to monitor her hemoglobin. She also accepted advice on stress management.

Billy had a torn diaphragm. He needed surgery to replace the stomach into the abdomen and to suture over the hole in his diaphragm. He was also warned about future macho challenges from his buddies!

Liz's pregnancy heartburn cured itself when the baby was born.

Peter's hernia was also managed at home without surgery. Keeping him upright allowed his esophagus, diaphragm, and stomach to develop normally.

From all of the above cases, it is clear that there are times when doctors must consider diagnoses other than hiatus hernia as a cause of the typical symptoms. This was touched upon in chapter 3, where esophageal disorders other than true hiatus hernia were discussed. Some diseases quite apart from esophageal disorders mimic the symptoms of hiatus hernia, and these are discussed in the next chapter.

Chapter 5

Ruling Out Other Causes

Some people with hiatus hernia panic when the symptoms get worse or when a new symptom appears. This is understandable; we all tend to regard any pain in the chest, for example, as angina pectoris—or even a heart attack—until it is proven otherwise. (*Angina pectoris* is chest pain that falls short of a full heart attack.) For others, the problem is the exact opposite: they assume, because they know they have a hiatus hernia, that it is the cause of any new symptom they experience, and they believe they have no need to worry. Ignoring new symptoms can be as bad for you as panicking unnecessarily, because this time the chest pain could be a heart attack—and if it is, you need to act quickly.

This chapter is therefore directed to both these groups—for want of better words, to both the panicky and the laid-back.

"Is It a Heart Attack?"

The pressing question for everyone with chest pain has to be: is it a heart attack? If you already know you have a hiatus hernia, then you are probably familiar with your particular type of chest pain. But what happens if it changes? What are the respective chances of the new pain being caused by heart trouble or by your hernia? And could the pain be due to something else—say, something in the lung or the stomach?

Let us look at how your doctor will approach the investigation of your chest pain. First, because failing to spot a heart attack has much more serious consequences than a delay in diagnosing esophagitis, all pain behind the breastbone (called *retrosternal* pain), whether or not it travels into the neck or arm, is presumed to come from the heart until proved otherwise.

Doctors cannot presume, simply because a retrosternal pain follows eating a large meal, that it is due to esophagitis. Eating is as likely to provoke angina in a susceptible person as it is to provoke esophageal pain in a person with a hiatus hernia—and coronary disease is more frequent in people with hiatus hernias than in the general population. It is quite common to suffer from both esophageal and coronary disease, and no matter how detailed the history taken by your doctor, he or she cannot make a definitive diagnosis without doing further tests to confirm or eliminate heart disease.

Therefore, if you have a new chest pain, even if you already know you have a hiatus hernia, you will be sent for cardiac investigations. These include a straight electrocardiogram (ECG), exercise ECG testing, echocardiogram, and if the evidence supports angina, coronary angiography. (All these tests are described in my book *Living with Angina*, published in the U.K. by Sheldon Press and in the U.S. by New Harbinger Publications.)

Some idea of how many cases of retrosternal chest pain are actually caused by esophageal problems, how many are due to coronary disease, and how the two can be differentiated was given by Drs. J. R. Bennett and M. Atkinson. In the 1980s, they studied 200 consecutive patients admitted to their hospital with such pain. In just under a quarter (23 percent) of the patients, the pain was coming from the esophagus alone. They found that the two groups of patients—those with heart disease and those with esophageal disease—tended to describe the quality of their pain in different ways.

Those who turned out to have heart disease spoke of their pain as "gripping," "vicelike," or "tight." Those who were found to have esophagitis complained of "burning." However, the differences could not be relied upon, because there was too much overlap in the descriptions between the two groups for a definitive diagnosis to be made on quality of pain alone.

The same applied to the distribution of the pain. Both patient groups admitted to feeling the pain in the neck, jaw, and arms. This was a surprise at the time of the study's publication, as until then doctors had assumed that pain radiating to the jaw and left arm was far more likely to come from the heart than the esophagus. Thirty years later, this Bennett/Atkinson finding is universally accepted.

Pain in the back—once held to more likely come from the esophagus than from the heart—was equally common in the two patient groups. Pain in the abdomen pointed more to esophageal disease than to heart disease, but as it was also a feature of some cases of angina, it was not a definitive sign of esophagitis.

The pain occurred more often with exercise in the heart patients and with changes in posture in the hiatus hernia patients. Breathlessness was more common in the heart patients, and regurgitation in those with hiatus hernia—but even these symptoms crossed over into the other diagnostic territories. Finally, Bennett and Atkinson stressed that chest pain may be the only symptom of esophageal disease such as hiatus hernia and that it may very closely mimic angina. This is particularly true of the nutcracker esophagus described in chapter 3 of this book.

"Could I Have Both Angina and Esophagitis?"

Unfortunately, the older we are, the more likely we are to have both angina and esophagitis. Dr. O. Svensson and his colleagues found that half of all their Swedish patients with coronary artery disease also had esophagitis, or disorders such as diffuse spasms or nutcracker esophagus.

Esophageal disorders have also been strongly linked with a

particular form of angina, Prinzmetal's angina, which is now thought to be caused by spasms of the muscles in the coronary arteries, rather than structural disease. Prinzmetal's angina, in contrast to classical angina, occurs when you are resting rather than taking exercise. Prinzmetal's angina attacks are caused when the muscles in the walls of the coronary arteries go into spasm—a mechanism similar to that of the diffuse spasm disorder of the esophagus described in chapter 3.

In two separate studies (by Drs. P. H. Ducrotte and E. L. Cattan and their colleagues) of patients with Prinzmetal's angina, 58 percent and 75 percent respectively also had disorders of esophageal spasm. The symptoms produced by coronary spasm and by esophageal spasm were indistinguishable, and their cause could only be identified by tests of heart and esophageal function, which are described in the next chapter.

In 1986, Dr. G. Vantrappen coined the term "irritable esophagus" for those people with pain exactly like angina but that actually stems from esophageal disease. In an article in *The Lancet*, he described thirty-three patients with such pain. Only twelve of them had an esophageal spasm without reflux of acid; the rest either combined spasms with reflux or had reflux alone. When he infused a small amount of acid into the esophagus of these patients, they all developed angina-like pain in the chest—exactly the pain for which they had been consulting their doctors. When they were taught how to avoid reflux (by using the self-treatment methods described in chapter 7), their pain disappeared.

In people with true angina, instilling acid into the esophagus has no pain-inducing effect, so this has been used as a test to differentiate between the two types of disease. True angina is more typically induced by exercise, which does not normally bring on esophageal pain. So if you are being investigated for central chest pain, do not be surprised if you are given both an exercise test and an acid-instillation test.

"Could My Symptoms Be Due to Gallbladder Problems?"

We have established that the symptoms of hiatus hernia include discomfort and a feeling of fullness in the upper abdomen after meals, heartburn, belching, and regurgitation of bitter fluid into the mouth. However, this array of symptoms also exactly describes what happens in gallbladder disease—in particular, chronic *chole-cystitis*, a long-standing inflammation of the gallbladder.

Why do the two conditions overlap so much? It appears that when the gallbladder is inflamed, this affects normal peristalsis at the overflow from the stomach to the duodenum, allowing bile and other digestive juices to run back up into the stomach. The mixture of the bile and the stomach's digestive juices irritates the cardia, and even if there is the smallest hiatus hernia (or even just an enlarged hiatus without a hernia), the backflow continues up into the esophagus.

Acid alone refluxing into the esophagus is bad enough—but with bile as well, the irritation to the lower esophagus is worse. Research scientists have added acid and bile, both together and separately, to pieces of human esophagus kept alive in culture. By far the most damage was done by the two together, but bile on its own, without acid, still caused considerable irritation. This may help to explain why some people do not respond completely to medicines aimed solely at reducing the impact of acid on the esophagus (see chapter 8 for a discussion of medicines).

The problem of experiencing both gallbladder trouble and reflux from the stomach into the esophagus is by no means rare. At least two British studies have shown that about half of the patients with gallbladder disease also had esophageal reflux. In another study (by J. R. Barker and J. Alexander-Williams), 34 percent of patients requiring surgery for gallbladder disease also had symptoms of esophageal reflux. Of those who were found during surgery to have an enlarged hiatus, more than 80 percent still experienced esophageal symptoms afterwards.

Barker and Alexander-Williams found that proportionately more women than men were cured of their symptoms by gallbladder removal and that the men and women with the most persistent symptoms after surgery were between ages forty and fifty-nine. It seems that patients who continue to experience symptoms after the gallbladder has been removed in fact suffered from two diseases: gallbladder disease and hiatus hernia. If the symptoms stop after surgery, then the main problem was gallbladder disease; in this case, the symptoms of reflux were a consequence of an irritated duodenum, stomach, and esophagus. Sadly, it sometimes takes removal of the gall bladder to find this out.

"Might I Have a Peptic Ulcer?"

Just as the symptoms of hiatus hernia and of gallbladder disease are difficult, if not impossible, to tell apart, so hiatus hernia can mimic duodenal and stomach ulcer symptoms, and vice versa. In some people with hiatus hernia, the pain is felt mainly in the upper abdomen and radiates to the back; this is identical to some peptic ulcer pain.

As with gallbladder disease, suffering from both a peptic ulcer and hiatus hernia is very common. British surgeons D. Flook and C. J. Stoddard showed that acid was entering the lower esophagus in 42 percent of their cases of duodenal ulcer, and R. Siewart found reflux in 40 percent of his duodenal ulcer patients. American R. J. Earlam and colleagues reported even higher figures: they saw microscopic evidence of esophagitis in twenty-five of their thirty-six patients with duodenal ulcers.

The experts are still arguing about why people with ulcers experience so much esophageal trouble. Some have suggested that the sphincter muscles in the cardia are faulty, and others blame minor degrees of hiatus hernia. The jury is still out. Suffice it to say that if you have a duodenal ulcer, it is best to assume that some of your symptoms are likely to come from esophageal reflux of acid, and you should treat yourself accordingly. How to do that is described in chapter 7.

"I Often Have Chest Complaints—Is This My Hernia, or Something Else As Well?"

I wrote in chapter 3 that many people with hiatus hernias also endure lung complications. This is because when they lie down (such as when they sleep), they inhale acid and other digestive juices that have flowed into the upper esophagus. Breathing in the contents of the esophagus can cause minor symptoms, such as hoarseness or a repeated cough, but it can also lead to bronchitis, pneumonia, and lung abscesses—all serious, and ultimately life-threatening, conditions.

It is easy to understand that lung problems can complicate severe esophagitis, but it appears that reflux does not need to be severe to create breathing problems. One study found that 40 percent of patients with what was classified as "benign esophageal disease" (meaning a small hiatus hernia without any chronic esophagitis or strictures) had lung problems directly due to their hiatus hernias. Many had asthma, a condition closely linked with esophagitis by other researchers.

The actual mechanism whereby so many people with hiatus hernias also experience breathing problems is not, however, as clear-cut as might be thought. Two groups of researchers found that in 4,000 scans of swallowing, only 2 percent of people with hiatus hernias actually breathed in their refluxed stomach contents. On the other hand, another study scanned nineteen patients overnight and found that five of them did so. It has been shown that many patients with reflux have laryngitis due to irritation of the upper esophagus—and if the acid regurgitation has reached the larynx, then it is very likely to have entered the lungs.

However, there is another explanation for the connection between hiatus hernias and lung disease. A nerve pathway exists (through the vagus nerve) that directly connects the esophagus and the main airways (the bronchi). Put a little acid into the lower end of the esophagus in a susceptible patient, and the bronchi will immediately constrict, causing an acute attack of asthmatic wheezing. There is no need for the patient actually to inhale any acid; the presence of acid in the lower esophagus is enough to set it off.

This is particularly true for asthmatic children. Dr. N. M. Wilson and colleagues made an overnight study of twenty children with asthma. They found that an asthma attack could be much more easily provoked when the children were lying flat and asleep, and that the attacks were associated with hiatus hernia and reflux of acid into the esophagus. The link has been proved, for when the hiatus hernia is repaired surgically in such children and their reflux stops, not only do their symptoms of esophagitis disappear, but so does their asthma. In these children, antireflux surgery was much more successful than the use of the acid-suppressant drug cimetidine (see chapter 8), but using both together has been found to be even better. In another study, cimetidine was given without surgery to asthmatic children with reflux due to hiatus hernia, and their asthma symptoms improved. The same may well be true for many adults.

"Could it Be Cancer?"

It is natural for people who have symptoms such as difficulty with swallowing, regurgitation, and central chest pain to fear that they may have cancer. It is true that cancers do occur in the esophagus and that they may or may not be linked with longstanding esophagitis due to reflux of acid. It is essential to understand when you should suspect that something other than a simple hiatus hernia may be causing your symptoms. If you do not take prompt action when such suspicions arise, you may be delaying any possible cure until it is too late.

The main symptom of an esophageal tumor is difficulty in swallowing. It does not, as a rule, cause heartburn or pain. The first symptom may arise suddenly, perhaps when trying to swallow a particularly large chunk of food, such as a fairly tough piece of meat that has not been completely chewed. Or it may come on gradually, so that swallowing becomes slower and the food seems to take longer going down than it used to. In the later stages, there is no pleasure in eating or drinking, and the patient loses weight because he or she is not taking in any food.

However, a sufferer should have consulted with his or her doctor long before that stage. Anyone who has any difficulty in swallowing should always see his or her doctor, who will always, in the first instance, refer the case to a specialist for X-rays and endoscopy of the swallowing mechanism.

Most of the time—and particularly when there are other symptoms of hiatus hernia, such as heartburn and symptoms caused by postural changes—the trouble is found to stem from a stricture. This is a narrowing of the esophagus due to old scar tissue, which in turn has been caused by years of exposure to acid (see chapters 3 and 4).

One relatively rare cause of difficulty with swallowing goes by at least three different names: it may be called *sideropenic dysphagia*, *Paterson-Brown-Kelly syndrome*, or *Plummer-Vinson syndrome*. (The name the doctor uses depends on which medical school he or she attended.) Whatever it is called, it affects women between thirty and sixty years old, and it has three features: severe anemia, a chronic inflammation of the tongue, and choking when trying to swallow solid food.

The swallowing difficulty in this condition starts because of esophageal spasm, which is limited to the upper half of the esophagus, but which eventually becomes a stricture, at which point the difficulty in swallowing grows much worse. On looking down the throat, a web can be seen stretched across it, at the level of the larynx. If this is neglected, cancer can develop in the area of this web, so it should be examined urgently. The treatment is to remove any stricture and to give iron to counter the anemia. Follow-up includes blood tests to ensure that the anemia is not returning and examinations to ensure that no malignant change is occurring.

Achalasia, strictures, and Patterson-Brown-Kelly syndrome

apart, swallowing difficulties may be caused by tumors in the esophagus.

Some esophageal tumors are benign *leiomyomas*: overgrowths of esophageal-wall muscle that project into the passage, interfering with the passing of food through its lower end. Leiomyomas are usually easily removed through an endoscope; an instrument to remove them can be passed down the flexible, hollow endoscope.

Cancers of the esophagus are a disease of older age: 75 percent of esophageal cancers occur in people over sixty. It attacks three times as many men as women. About half of all cancers of the esophagus arise in the middle third of its length, and about 30 percent in its lower third, suggesting to most experts that constant exposure to reflux of acid from the stomach may contribute to the cause. (Although the lower third is more exposed to acid, the middle third is thought to be more sensitive to acid-provoked cancerous changes.) So repairing a hiatus hernia and stopping the esophagus from being awash with acid may well prevent many cancers—a good reason for sticking strictly to your doctor's advice and treatment. This is particularly true if you have a Barrett's esophagus (see chapter 3), which is associated with a higher than normal incidence of cancer.

Proof that looking after yourself may, by curing esophagitis, prevent cancer is suggested in a study by R. Kuylenstierna and E. Munch-Wickland, published in the *Journal of Cancer* in 1985. They reviewed the case histories of 163 patients with esophageal cancer; 10 percent of them had had esophagitis. Of the 51 patients with lower-esophageal cancer, 13 (25 percent) had had esophagitis. There were no cases of esophagitis among the 47 with upper-esophageal cancer; the other 65 had cancer of the middle third of the esophagus. It seems clear from these figures that chronic esophagitis can precede cancer of the lower esophagus if it is not kept under control or, preferably, eradicated.

This whole chapter can be summarized in a few sentences. Hiatus hernia and esophagitis are inextricably linked and give rise to many different symptoms and collections of symptoms. These can be confused with the symptoms of other conditions, such as heart disease, gallbladder disease, peptic ulcers, bronchitis and asthma, and cancer. Making a definitive diagnosis of hiatus hernia with reflux and esophagitis is often (almost always, in fact) impossible without conducting some tests. So if you are seeing your doctor for the first time with symptoms typical of hiatus hernia, you will almost certainly be referred to a gastroenterological clinic for such tests.

These tests and the reasons for them are described in the next chapter.

Chapter 6

Tests for Hiatus Hernia and Reflux

Once your doctor suspects you have a hiatus hernia, he or she will make one of two decisions: either to make a diagnosis on the basis of what you have told him or her (following a brief examination) or to ask a specialist—a gastroenterologist—to conduct further tests.

If your diagnosis is made without a referral to a specialist, your doctor is not neglecting you. The tests take much time and are very expensive, so if the diagnosis can be made from the symptoms alone, this is a great savings. In these times of health costs rapidly spiraling upwards, such savings are vital. Doing without tests also allows treatment to be started earlier, and if the symptoms respond to the initial treatment, this is in effect a practical confirmation of the diagnosis. Doing without tests is also much more pleasant for the patient, as some of the tests can be uncomfortable, even distressing.

Symptom-Score Systems

However, any diagnosis, even one made from symptoms alone, should be based on objective judgement rather than vague hunch. Several groups of gastroenterologists have therefore set up symptom-score systems to determine the severity of the condition and how they might best manage it.

Here it must be said that the most important aim of investigating hiatus hernia symptoms is not to find out the size of the hernia (one can have a large hernia without symptoms, while a small hernia can cause huge problems). Instead, the priority is to determine the severity of the esophagitis caused by the hernia and the best way to reverse its effects. It is the esophagitis, after all, that causes the heartburn and pain and that can lead to future esophageal ulcers, strictures, bleeding, and even perforation.

The aim is to cure the esophagitis. If that means simply protecting the esophagus from acid, then so be it. If it means surgery to repair the hernia and therefore to stop the reflux of acid into the esophagus, then that must also be decided upon. The symptom scores are therefore a measure of esophagitis, rather than of the hernia itself, and they help the doctor decide how to treat a particular patient.

Table 6.1: Scoring System for Symptoms of Esophagitis

(from DeMeester et al.)

Symptom	Grade	Description
Heartburn		
None	0	No heartburn
Mild	1	Occasional episodes
Moderate	2	Reason for visit to doctor
Severe	3	Enough to interfere with daily life
Regurgitation		
None	0	No regurgitation
Mild	1	Occasional episodes
Moderate	2	Predictable on moving position or straining
Severe	3	Associated with nighttime cough or pneumonia
Swallowing difficulty (dysphagia)		
None	0	No dysphagia
Mild	1	Occasional episodes
Moderate	2	Needs a drink to clear it
Severe	3	At least one episode of obstruction needing medical treatment

Table 6.2: Scoring System for Esophagitis

(from Jamieson and Duranceau)

	One point	Two points	Three points	Four points
Frequency	Less than once a month	More often than once a month, but less often than weekly	More often than once a week, but less often than daily	Every day
Duration	Less than 6 months	More than 6 months; less than 24 months	More than 24 months; less than 60 months	More than 60 months
Severity	Nuisance value only	Spoils enjoyment of life	Interferes with living normally	Worst possible symptoms

The score for frequency is added to that for duration, and the sum is multiplied by that for severity. This gives a minimum score for each symptom of 2 and a maximum of 32; the case is classified as mild if the score is from 1–7, moderate 8–15, marked 16–23, and severe 24–32.

Two scoring systems are in general use. The first was developed by Dr. T. R. DeMeester and his colleagues (see Table 6.1). It lists three separate symptoms of esophagitis and grades each of them according to its severity on a scale of 0 to 3 points. The grades are very specifically described, resulting in similar scores for people with a similar severity of disease. This is important not just so that treatment can be decided on a standard assessment, but also so that clinical trials of new treatments can be fairly assessed and the results subjected to good statistical evaluation.

An alternative to this system was developed by Drs. G. G. Jamieson and A. C. Duranceau. They assigned to each symptom a series of points according to the severity, frequency, and duration of symptoms. The higher the score, the more severe the problem. Table 6.2 shows how this system works.

The system can be used for each symptom (heartburn; swallowing difficulties including pain, regurgitation, bleeding, and chest problems); the scores for each symptom are added together to give an overall score.

Once the history has been taken, the examination completed, and the provisional diagnosis made, the next step (if the decision is made to investigate further rather than simply to start treatment) is to plan the tests to be done.

The tests measure four areas of esophageal function:

* its ability to swallow;

* the presence of any refluxed stomach material;

* any damage to the inner layer of esophageal lining;

* the response of the lowest part of the esophagus to acid.

The tests include X-rays, endoscopies, biopsies, and other tests to assess the esophageal physiology (such as manometry to assess the pressure within the esophagus). These are all described below.

X-Ray Tests

X-ray examination is usually the first test. A straight X-ray of the chest can sometimes show a gas bubble within the stomach, well above the diaphragm, confirming a hiatus hernia—but this can be difficult to see and depends on the presence of air in the stomach at the time of the X-ray. So "contrast" X-rays are used to make things much clearer.

The usual technique involves a barium drink, which the patient swallows while the radiologist watches the moving film. The changing shape of the lump of barium passing down the esophagus can show problems of mobility (such as achalasia and spasm), the presence of reflux through the cardia, and even inflammation in the lower esophagus. Such barium-swallows have shown that many patients with reflux esophagitis also experience a much slower clearance of barium from the lower end of the esophagus into the stomach.

However, a barium-swallow alone is not always a reliable indicator of reflux and esophagitis. For example, one study revealed a reflux during a barium-swallow in 20 percent of patients who were later found not to have any esophagitis; the same study showed no reflux in 35 percent of people who had moderate and severe esophagitis. To make the test more accurate, another study looked at the reflux produced when patients lay on their left side and were given the barium and some water to drink. They were then asked to turn to their right sides and were given some food (bread and paté). The aim of this step was to expose the maximum opening of the cardia, from the stomach back into the esophagus, to the pressures of both food and gravity. If reflux occurs, it should show in this position. This study found a connection between reflux and esophagitis in fifteen out of twenty-six patients with symptoms. In all, twenty had food-stimulated reflux, and twenty-three had esophagitis.

Do not be surprised, therefore, if during your barium-swallow you are moved around from side to side: your radiologist is trying to see if you experience any reflux. If you do, its extent will be graded by how far it travels up your esophagus—and your treatment will be planned accordingly.

Two refinements on the usual barium-swallow have been introduced in the last few years. One is a double-contrast technique, which involves the patient's swallowing some barium very quickly; the esophagus is then distended with gas from a fizzy powder (or from swallowing air). In the other technique, you are asked first to swallow about a tablespoon of alkaline solution, then about half a cup of barium, a tablespoon of an acid solution, and three drops of a "bubble breaker." This shows the lining of the lower esophagus in great detail, even to the extent of highlighting small ulcers in its surface. It gives the radiologist a very accurate picture of how much reflux there is and the extent of the damage it has done to the esophagus. Both of these techniques have shown that many people have a hiatus hernia without actually having esophagitis; they also indicate that patients with esophagitis almost always have a hiatus hernia, with acid flowing freely back through the cardia.

Endoscopy and Biopsy

The flexible fiber-optic *endoscope* has made a huge contribution to our knowledge of medicine in recent years, and nowhere more so than in the investigation of hiatus hernias and esophagitis. An endoscope is a fully flexible tube through which runs a bundle of glass fibers. The operator can see very clearly through the endo-scope what is going on inside the throat, esophagus, and stomach. It also allows instruments to be passed along its length so that biopsies (pieces of tissue) can be taken for tests, in full view of the operator.

The endoscope is passed, under local anesthetic, into the esophagus. It may sound horrendous to endure such a procedure without a general anesthetic, but the sedative makes you so drowsy that you hardly feel the discomfort and will have very little memory of it afterwards.

Endoscopy gives its operator a clear, magnified view of what is happening over the whole length of the esophagus, the cardia, and the stomach. It is used for diagnosis, to assess the severity and extent of esophagitis, and for biopsies (explained below). An endoscopy can also be used to relate the site of the cardia (the junction between esophagus and stomach) to the level of the diaphragm; this site is clearly seen as the Z-line, a sharp difference in appearance of the surface as esophageal tissue becomes stomach tissue.

Endoscopy is a relatively young technique, so it is not surpris-ing that experts still disagree on how to assess the severity of esophagitis. They have, however, partly agreed on a classification of esophagitis, which helps them to decide on how to proceed with treatment. Grade I esophagitis means that the only sign of inflam-mation is some redness and a little friability. Grade II indicates the presence of some superficial ulcers (something like mouth ulcers).

Grades III and IV show many more, and deeper, ulcers, with strictures or shortening. Barrett's esophagus is Grade IV.

As a rule of thumb, people with the lower grades of esophagitis are usually given medical (rather than surgical) treatment; those with higher grades are at more risk of bleeding and other complications and are likely to be treated more intensively with more powerful drugs and to be seen more often. Patients who have a hiatus hernia along with higher-grade esophagitis (which is usually the case) will be scheduled for surgery to repair it on an urgent basis.

Just looking at the esophageal lining sometimes fails to give a definitive diagnosis; biopsies to confirm inflammation at the microscopic level may be needed. This means that the endoscope is adapted to take several tiny pieces of tissue from different suspicious-looking areas at each endoscopy session. Taking biopsies does not cause pain. Scientists have agreed on the microscopic appearances that confirm esophagitis in a biopsy sample, so taken together, the appearance of the esophagus through an endoscope and the appearance of a biopsy sample through a microscope make for a very accurate diagnosis.

Manometry: Measuring Pressures

Not all hiatus hernia sufferers have esophagitis. The case histories in chapter 1 show that the problem for some is not heartburn, but pain from esophageal spasm or from the bulk of a rolling hernia in the chest. Through an endoscope such cases look normal. But the pressures inside the esophagus during spasms, or when the herniated stomach is full of food or gas, can be very abnormal. Measuring these pressure swings can be a great help both in diagnosis and in assessing treatment.

To investigate such patients, *manometry* (pressure measurement) is of great value. There are two systems; both use thin catheters (one system uses a hollow tube, the other a solid tube), which are passed through the nose into the esophagus and stomach. Both systems measure the pressures above, within, and below the sphincter, as well as the pressure waves produced in peristalsis.

Although manometry is ineffective in diagnosing esophagitis, it can establish that a patient suffers from one of the muscle (or motility) disorders, such as achalasia, diffuse spasm, or nutcracker esophagus. However, a single patient can have both types of esophageal disorder. In one study of 102 patients with diagnosed esophageal acid reflux due to hiatus hernia, manometry showed that 6 also had achalasia, 4 had diffuse spasm, and 2 had a nutcracker esophagus. When planning treatment, whether surgical or medical, it is important to take both conditions into account; surgery to repair a hernia in such patients may not cure their symptoms.

It must be said here that manometry is a very specialized investigation that will always be confined to a small proportion of patients with particular problems. The same can be said of the next investigations, provocation tests.

Provocation Tests

Sometimes the description of a symptom such as heartburn is unusual. It may not be described as burning, it may appear in an unusual place, or it may not relate to food or hunger—yet the doctor may suspect that it is caused by acid reflux from stomach to esophagus. In any of these cases, an acid provocation test may be carried out.

Its aim is simply to see whether putting a little acid into the lower esophagus provokes the symptom of which the patient is complaining. That is not as bad as it sounds, as only a little acid is used, and many precautions are taken to ensure that no damage is done.

The Bernstein Test

Three provocation tests are in current use: the Bernstein test, the acid clearance test, and the standard acid reflux test. As with other aspects of hiatus hernia investigations and diagnosis, the experts do not agree on their relative usefulness.

In the Bernstein test, the patient sits in a chair while a thin catheter is passed through the nostril down into the lower esophagus. As with all such catheter tests, the patient may choke a little as the end passes the larynx, but once the tube is in place, the patient hardly notices it. Once the patient is settled and the catheter is in place, a little saline (salt solution) is passed through the catheter for about fifteen minutes. At some point after this, without the patient's being told when, the saline is replaced by an acid solution for about thirty minutes. If the symptoms do not appear during this time, it can be assumed that they are not caused by acid reflux. If they do appear, the acid is immediately replaced by saline. This usually relieves the pain quite quickly, at least within twenty minutes. Only a few people report that the pain lasts longer. As soon as the test is finished, the patient is given an antacid.

A positive Bernstein test shows only that the esophagus is sensitive to acid; its main use is to help sort out the cause of a pain in patients whose symptoms are not the run-of-the-mill sort typical of esophagitis or hiatus hernia.

The Acid Clearance Test

The acid clearance test is also performed with the patient in a sitting position. Usually carried out just after manometry, it is done with the pressure-measuring catheter still in place. The patient is asked to swallow another fine tube, this time with an acid-measuring electrode at the end. A little acid is passed into the lower end of the esophagus through the manometry catheter, and the patient is asked to swallow every thirty seconds until the acid no longer registers with the electrode. The acid clears after three swallows in normal subjects; it can take many more swallows in people with esophagitis.

The Acid Reflux Test

The standard acid reflux test measures whether the patient can prevent acid that has been introduced into the stomach from entering the esophagus. This time, acid is put into the stomach via a catheter, and readings from the acid-measuring electrode are taken on either side of the cardia. In people with no reflux, the acid disappears less than one centimeter above the cardia; in people who have reflux, the acid still registers some distance up into the lower esophagus. During the test the patient is asked to cough, to take deep breaths, and to strain as if he is lifting a heavy weight—all in four positions. The test is positive if acid passes into the esophagus on at least two occasions in the 20 tests and positions. This test identifies people with moderate to severe reflux, but it can only be used along with the results of the other examinations as a guide to treatment; it is not accurate enough to be used alone.

Acid Monitoring

Because the results of the above tests are less reliable than we would wish, many gastroenterologists now use pH monitoring as the main test for acid reflux. The pH scale measures acidity and alkalinity; it ranges from less than 1 (extremely acid) to just under 14 (extremely alkaline), with neutral being a pH of 7.

The technology of pH monitoring is changing very fast, so what I write about pH sensors may well become out of date by the time this book is published. However, the principles remain the same. The aim is to leave a pH monitor in the lower esophagus for eighteen to twenty-four hours; it records everything happening during that time. One system uses radio telemetry, allowing the patient to go home, so the pH changes can be recorded during normal, everyday life.

As with other aspects of hiatus hernia and its complications, the experts disagree on what constitutes abnormality and its severity. Most feel that a pH of 4 or less in the esophagus is abnormal, but debate continues as to how long it should remain at that level, and under what circumstances, before it is considered serious. However, "normal" levels have been established: in Professor Alfred Cuschieri's unit in Dundee, Scotland, twenty-four-hour pH monitoring of 50 volunteers with no symptoms showed very few occurrences of a pH below 4, especially when they were lying down, and extremely few of those occurrences lasted for five minutes or more.

The most sensitive test for assessment of reflux is twenty-four-hour pH monitoring. Shortened to 12 hours, the test is still reasonably accurate, and many hospital departments have shortened it even further, to the three hours after a meal, with little if any further loss of accuracy. The shorter tests are cheaper and more convenient, but the twenty-four-hour test remains, according to Professor Cuschieri, the "gold standard" because it traces the evolution of reflux over a whole, typical day and night.

A monitoring test of eighteen to twenty-four hours has proved very useful in children. Tiny electrodes are used, and most children tolerate it reasonably well, considering that it involves inserting tubes down the throat. American pediatric gastroenterologists have shown that such a test is a reliable basis for deciding upon surgery in infants.

Radio-Isotope Scans

The newest test involves asking the patient to swallow material containing a tiny amount of radiation and following what happens with a "gamma camera" as the food is propelled down the esophagus into the stomach. The patient sits upright and chews a teaspoonful of poached egg white in which there is a tiny amount of radioactive technetium (a substance that very rapidly loses its radioactivity, so it can do no harm).

The patient then swallows the egg white in a single gulp and continues to swallow every twenty seconds thereafter. The gamma camera records what is going on for four minutes. The time it takes for all the egg to pass into the stomach is less than fifteen seconds in a normal esophagus; it can take much longer in patients with a hiatus hernia. From this test, Professor Cuschieri's team has identified five different patterns of food passage down the esophagus and into the stomach and can relate the patterns to the clinical symptoms. One of these patterns, of course, is normal. Other patients show:

* oscillation, in which the egg white bounces down and up the esophagus;

* nonclearance, in which the egg white fails to enter the stomach within the four minutes;

* step-delay, in which it is held up in the middle or lower third of the esophagus;

* nonspecific, in which the flow is abnormal, but does not fit into a particular pattern.

Oscillation is the typical pattern in achalasia, and Professor Cuschieri recommends this test for screening patients suspected of having this or one of the related esophageal motility disorders.

Radio-isotope scans are often used for children, in which case the material is administered in fruit juice or milk, and the scan continues for up to an hour. As there is no tube to be swallowed or inserted, children tolerate it much better than the other tests, so it is being increasingly used in children as a screening test prior to making a treatment decision.

Treatment for both children and adults involves three aspects: management of one's own lifestyle, medication, and surgery. They will be discussed in the next three chapters.

Chapter 7

Managing Your Own Hiatus Hernia

The firm aim of all treatment for hiatus hernia is to reduce the symptoms. Whether these are caused by esophagitis, leading to heartburn and regurgitation, or by the presence of a large mass of stomach in the chest, leading to pain, bloating, and swallowing difficulties, the need is the same: to keep the stomach and cardia below the diaphragm and to minimize the possibilities for reflux.

This needs an effort from you as well as from your doctors. You need to understand what to avoid and how to promote a healthier relationship between your esophagus, diaphragm, and stomach. Making a real difference may require several changes—some drastic—in your lifestyle.

Posture, Position, and Keeping Fit

First and foremost, you must avoid postures and actions that cause reflux and increase the size of the hernia through the hiatus. Above all, this means avoiding any action that increases the pressure inside the abdomen, pushing the cardia up through the hiatus. Bending over is the obvious action that must be avoided. When you bend, your abdominal-wall muscles contract, increasing the pressure inside the abdominal cavity. Especially if you have a larger hiatus than normal, increased abdominal pressure can force the upper part of the stomach through the diaphragm into the chest, thereby flooding the lower esophagus with acid. Heartburn will inevitably occur under such circumstances.

So, until your hiatus hernia is mended and your esophagitis has healed, do not bend over. This is a good excuse to postpone all those awkward jobs you don't really like, such as weeding the garden or clearing out bottom drawers. But it also rules out some sports, such as bowling or curling.

Other activities besides postural changes also cause the abdominal muscles to contract (and thus further damage the esophagus). Some additional activities to avoid include: lifting heavy weights (such as bags of groceries or bundles of logs), pushing a loaded wheelbarrow or a lawnmower, shoveling snow, and chopping wood. Straining to pass a constipated stool is yet another, so modify your diet (if necessary) to keep your bowel movements regular and your stools soft. Doing weight-training or weight-lifting, including sit-ups or stomach crunches, can also create problems. And any explosive sport, such as those involving throwing or hitting a ball (which increase the pressure inside the abdomen when we hit a ball while holding our breath), can set off symptoms.

Keeping fit is highly recommended, but do so by participating only in exercises that keep you breathing steadily, such as walking, running, and dancing. If you can swim in a semi-upright position (that is, by doggie paddling), then swimming is fine, but any of the regulation strokes, which all require a horizontal position, should be avoided, and by all means avoid doing the sidestroke on your right side. Diving is not recommended. Cycling is fine, as long as you ride a bike that doesn't require crouching over the handlebars.

Lying down, even with the abdominal muscles relaxed, can promote a backflow of acid into the esophagus or, in a rolling hernia, the displacement of the stomach upwards—so try to keep the chest above the abdomen at all times, even when sleeping. If you have only a mild hiatus hernia with few symptoms, all you may need is an extra pillow or two. If you find this is not enough, then try the blocks under the foot of the bed and a pillow support as described in chapter 4. If you put blocks under the head of the bed, make sure you can't slip down toward the foot of the bed when sleeping.

Eating

How you eat matters more than *what* you eat. In the past, people with hiatus hernias were advised to eat various weird and wonderful diets, the main components of which were milk, crackers, and steamed white fish. There was absolutely no scientific basis for these diets—all they did was tend to make things worse by causing sufferers (from the diet, that is!) to gain weight. People were also advised not to eat or drink acidic foods, such as citrus fruits and juices. This was a complete misunderstanding of digestion; the acid in our stomachs does not relate in any way to the amount of fruit of any kind that we eat.

It is important, however, to time your meals correctly and to eat the correct quantities at each meal. If you eat a small amount every two hours, your stomach settles down to produce a small, constant amount of acid throughout the day. This acid is used up in digesting your small meals. This regimen is far less likely to provoke esophagitis than the usual three large meals a day, which stimulate the stomach to secrete large volumes of acid and pepsin, much of which can overflow into the esophagus.

In addition, the larger the volume of food you pack into your stomach, the more likely it is to be displaced up into your chest, especially if you feel drowsy afterwards and decide to put your feet up. On the other hand, don't go to bed at night on a completely empty stomach: a small glass of milk and a few crackers can help to neutralize any acid produced during the first few hours of sleeping. Don't eat or drink any more than this. A larger meal just before lying down (or for that matter just before exercise) is likely to promote symptoms by distending the stomach and increasing the pressure within it. This can lead to regurgitation of food through the cardia into the esophagus—the last thing you need at night.

If you do believe that a particular item of food causes pain, then avoid that food. However, there is no reason to follow faddish diets or to restrict what you eat generally. Keep in mind that everyone needs to eat a wide range of foods with the proper amounts of fats, carbohydrates, proteins, vitamins, minerals, and water to remain healthy and that many restricted diets are deficient in one or another of these important components.

Obesity

Equally important is following good advice about weight management. Do not let yourself become overweight, and if you are overweight, lose the extra pounds. Many sufferers of hiatus hernia are several—or many—pounds overweight; they often lose their symptoms completely when they return to the normal weight for their height.

This is particularly true of those who have a tendency toward being "apple-shaped" rather than "pear-shaped." Apple-shaped people put on extra fat around the middle; pear-shaped people have big bottoms and hips. In those who are apple-shaped, much of the fat accumulates inside the abdomen and competes with the stomach for room. Especially if the hiatus is larger than normal, the extra abdominal fat pushes the stomach up and through it. Shedding the extra fat allows room for the stomach to find its proper place. However, those who are pear-shaped should not let this information make them complacent. Pear-shaped obese people often find that losing weight helps their hiatus hernia symptoms enormously. Why this occurs is less understood, but suffice it to say that the reason for the improvement does not matter so much as the result.

Losing weight is not easy for anyone, but it is more difficult for hiatus hernia sufferers than most, because they often find that eating dairy products and crackers or cookies is the best way to ease pain. Unfortunately, these foods also happen to be full of fat-inducing calories. If you are overweight and find yourself going for the fridge each time you feel pain, make a diversion instead towards the medicine cabinet and take a little antacid instead of milk. Once you start losing weight you should find yourself making fewer trips to either destination.

The best way to lose weight is to eat a little less of what you normally eat, to eat a balanced diet, and to exercise a little more in a way that you enjoy. Don't try any crash diets; they never work permanently because no one sticks to them for very long, and most crash dieters have a massive rebound to an even higher weight than before. In addition, the irregular meals and imbalanced eating that characterize many fad diets can increase the amount of acid in the stomach—and thus worsen your esophagitis. And be wary of buying a fancy new exercise machine. Very few people have the discipline to keep using one at home on their own. It is a good idea to join a weight-loss group. Surrounding yourself with like-minded people can help you gain confidence and make friends while you lose weight.

Drinking and Smoking

The oldest medical cliche is that we can keep healthy if we do everything in moderation. Sadly, this just isn't so for people with hiatus hernia who like a drink and a smoke!

Alcohol relaxes the cardia, so it can actually promote reflux. In the form of hard liquor, it directly irritates the lower esophagus, especially one affected by esophagitis. So avoid hard liquor completely. Remember that this advice comes from a Scot living in a whisky-distilling district, so it is given only after much deliberation and even anguish! The good news is that wines and beers are less likely to be a problem, as long as they are restricted to a glass or two in any one day. If you are drinking up to the legal limit for driving (which in any case is too high), you are probably drinking too much.

I have no such good news for cigarette smokers—or users of tobacco in any form. If you smoke only one cigarette per day, that is one too many. Dozens of reasons exist for not smoking—among them the annual 400,000-plus early deaths in the United States directly attributable to tobacco use—and they certainly apply to hiatus hernia sufferers.

To start with, tobacco use lowers the pressure across the cardia, so it causes more reflux. Secondly, it directly irritates the esophageal surface, so it worsens esophagitis. If these reasons were not enough, it also delays the healing of any ulcer, so it can make bleeding and perforation more likely—especially in severe cases, such as Barrett's esophagus. Finally, tobacco use promotes cancer, so it is a crazy habit for people in whom the risk is already raised, however slightly, because they suffer from esophagitis or a Barrett's esophagus.

Quitting Your Tobacco Habit

If you have encountered difficulty in quitting smoking, or if you believe that the warnings against tobacco use do not apply to you, or if you feel willing to continue taking the risk, then mull over the next few paragraphs. If you heed them, they may save your life.

In the 1980s I, like many other doctors at the time, advised people that they could stop smoking in one of two ways. They could do it gradually, over several weeks, or they could stop suddenly, all at once. Now I'm convinced that the latter is by far the better way.

Quitting cold turkey is sometimes called the General de Gaulle method, because Charles de Gaulle announced on television to the whole French nation that he had stopped smoking. After that, he could hardly light up in case a member of the press or a political opponent saw him and exposed him as a fraud or a backslider. Most of us could use a similar method. We may not be as famous as the general, but we all have a circle of friends whose respect we wish to keep. We could announce our resolve to them and enlist their aid in helping us stick to our good intentions.

Today, the antismoking climate will ensure their sympathy and support rather than their sneers or sniggers.

I advise people to locate all the cigarettes they possess—in pockets and handbags, at home and elsewhere—and to tear them up and throw them in the trash or on the fire. They should resolve never to buy another cigarette and always to say no immediately, without even thinking about it, to anyone who offers them one. If they do not wish to argue with their friends who smoke, no-smoking signs posted conspicuously in the car and at home can help.

People who contemplate quitting cold turkey often fear withdrawal symptoms, such as agitation, irritability, sleeplessness, and nervousness. They do not need to; often there are no withdrawal symptoms. People who must give up smoking for serious medical reasons, such as lung cancer or heart disease, rarely experience withdrawal symptoms, probably because they realize the serious consequences of continuing. The same applies to anyone with hiatus hernia and esophagitis, and particularly with Barrett's esophagus. For these patients, smoking can kill—through an ulcer that bleeds or becomes perforated or because chronic esophagitis has turned into cancer. These are as serious as health problems can get, and once this truth hits home, smokers usually find it easy to stop.

Once you quit, you may still have the desire to smoke. But that will subside before long, and your new feeling of well-being, caused by the elimination from your body of carbon monoxide, nicotine, and tars, will take over. You may also experience much less pain from your esophagitis as the raw esophageal lining begins to heal. If you need something to help take your mind off cigarettes, chew sugar-free gum or munch on carrots and celery. Get friends to support you in your efforts. If you can't stop the first time, try again. Many people find that they must quit several times before they manage to do so permanently. Try acupuncture or hypnotherapy if you wish. Although these techniques do not offer any magical properties, some people find them helpful, and as I've stated before, a successful result is more important than the reason behind the success.

Sufferers of hiatus hernia should avoid nicotine chewing gum or nicotine patches. These keep up the supply of nicotine to the irritated esophagitis, and nicotine is the very agent in tobacco that prevents healing. It is a powerful constrictor of arteries, and good blood flow to the esophagus is necessary for healing.

While quitting, a good viewpoint to adopt is to understand that over the years, you have used smoking as a crutch in times of stress. Obviously, it is not a helpful crutch, because it in no way changes the cause of your stress. So, if you must, replace smoking with another crutch—one that could be beneficial to your health. This can be anything, even starting to enjoy fruit again. Most smokers do not enjoy eating fruits and vegetables because their taste buds are so damaged from the smoke. When you stop smoking, your sense of taste comes alive again, and you can expand the variety of foods you enjoy eating. This will not only benefit your general health but will help your esophagus to heal too.

This is an ideal time to take up a new hobby and meet new friends. If you have been a regular smoker, your usual haunts are likely to have a smoky atmosphere, so change your social life. Avoid places where most people smoke, and be on guard against the offer of that first cigarette. One quickly leads to another, and you will soon be on the track to repeated esophagitis and chest pain. You will have to worry once again about whether the chest pain is coming from your hiatus hernia or from your heart—a worry that to a great extent could have been avoided.

If you have esophagitis and you smoke, you owe it to yourself and your family to stop. Take heart from the fact that you are not alone. Several million Americans have given up tobacco over the last several decades. According to the National Center for Chronic Disease Prevention and Health Promotion of the Centers for Disease Control and Prevention, fewer than 30 percent of U.S. adults now smoke. By stopping, you are simply joining the sensible majority. You are also making important positive changes in your own physiology.

Here is a list of the practical benefits of stopping smoking. It may help you in your resolve!

Within twenty minutes of stopping:

* Your blood pressure decreases to the normal range;

* Your pulse slows down to the normal rate;

* The circulation in your fingers and toes and in your esophagus begins to open up.

After eight hours:

* Carbon monoxide levels in the blood return to normal;

* Oxygen levels in the blood return to normal.

After one day:

* Your chances of heart attack have already diminished.

After two days:

* Your senses of smell and taste are heightened;

* Your coronary arteries are much wider;

* There is much better blood flow to your esophagus;

* Your blood is much less likely to clot.

After three days:

* Your airways have opened up;

* You are breathing more easily;

* Your heart is more efficient and less strained.

After two weeks to three months:

* Walking is easier;

* You can exercise for much longer;

* Your circulation is much improved.

After nine months:

* Your lungs are free of tars;

* You no longer have a morning cough.

After five years:

* Your risk of death from lung cancer has dropped from 137 to 72 per 100,000.

After ten years:

* Your risk of death from lung cancer has dropped to 12 per 100,000;

* You are at much less risk of dying from cancer of the mouth, pharynx, esophagus, bladder, kidney, or pancreas.

Surely, if you have been a smoker until now, these facts will persuade you to stop. So enjoy the fact that you are now a non-smoker. By making that decision, you have probably prolonged your life by many years.

Stress

No medical subject is more difficult to tackle than stress. Stress is blamed for a host of illnesses and symptoms, including heart attacks, strokes, stomach ulcers, asthma, skin complaints, and even cancer. People with proven hiatus hernias often feel worse when they are anxious or "keyed up" with a problem at work or in the home. Yet many good scientific studies have failed to confirm a direct link between either acute stress (the stress you feel in the "heat of the moment") or chronic stress (the tension caused by ongoing, unsolved problems) and the symptoms of indigestion, including heartburn. This may be because the studies can't pinpoint stress accurately enough. Stress is incredibly difficult to define and to measure. No matter how stressed we feel, in trials it doesn't show up as an increase in blood pressure or heart rate or stomach-acid output. Nor does it seem to affect the area most involved in hiatus hernia: the junction between the esophagus and the stomach.

Yet if we are to propose a direct link between stress and the worsening of symptoms of hiatus hernia, there must be a physical explanation for it. The link could be a stress-induced increase in pressure inside the stomach, pushing the stomach contents up into the chest. It could be a relaxation of the diaphragm or a lowering of the esophageal sphincter, allowing backflow of gastric juices into the esophagus. It could be an excessive secretion of stomach acids and digestive juices, which are more corrosive in someone who already has reflux into the chest.

None of these features are easily measurable in scientific studies, which could be why such studies have failed to make the expected connection between stress and hiatus hernia symptoms. But they could easily happen in everyday life. Under stress we become physically more tense; contracted stomach muscles could easily raise the pressure inside the abdomen, which, as we've discussed, can push the stomach further up into the chest. Worry can cause the stomach to oversecrete its digestive juices, and if we don't eat properly—another consequence of worry—there is nothing inside the stomach to neutralize the juices, and they start to digest the lower esophagus instead.

Emotional upsets can alter the tension in our gut (the phrase "stomach churning" comes immediately to mind). This can cause the sphincters to relax abnormally, and the stomach and gut muscles can go into overdrive, both forwards and in reverse. Their contents can be driven upward—as well as in the normal downward direction—and indigestion and heartburn can result.

On top of all this, our usual stress-relieving behaviors might make the problems worse! We might smoke more, which increases our stomach-acid output and makes us even more tense (it is a fallacy that smoking relaxes you; nicotine is a stimulant). Or maybe we cope by tending to reach for the bottle; alcohol irritates, rather than soothes, the stomach. We may even throw a temper tantrum, raising our blood pressure and intra-abdominal pressure when we do so. Throwing yourself on the floor and biting the carpet while foaming at the mouth will guarantee an indigestion attack!

So although stress is not the initial cause of hiatus hernia, the way we react to stress can make its symptoms worse. If we recognize this, we are halfway to dealing with it. If we can change the way we react to the stresses in our lives, we may be able to minimize the symptoms of hiatus hernia.

But how can we change the way we react to stress? The first trick is to adopt a good mental response to the emotional and physical stresses we face. This may require good psychological guidance, not necessarily from a professional "shrink," but at least from someone who knows you and your problems well and who has experience in dealing with emotions and anxieties. Your family doctor is a good start, and he or she may guide you to other advisors.

Second, analyze the cause of your stress and work to change it. If your stress is caused by some aspect of your job, begin steps to alter the situation. If your stress comes from people in your life, face them individually and sort out the problems. Learn skills for dealing with interpersonal problems amicably but firmly, while avoiding arguing (which will only produce more stress).

Third, put the cause of your stress into perspective. Is it really so much to worry about? Does it really affect your life so much? Is it worth ruining your health over? Answer these questions, preferably with your partner or a trusted friend. You may find that bringing fears out into the open can dispel them or at least give you a way to *start* dispelling them.

Finally, take time to relax. Every day, find some time to shrug off your worries completely. You may find release of stress in exercise, or in just listening to music. Some people take up yoga or transcendental meditation or attend relaxation classes; others find it just as helpful to relax in their own homes. Whatever works best for you, do it. And keep on doing it. You only have one life, so don't spend all of it on the treadmill. Step off every day for an hour or two; that by itself may ease your symptoms a lot.

If self-management alone proves insufficient to entirely clear your symptoms, the next chapter explains how medical treatment can help further.

Chapter 8

Medical Treatment of Hiatus Hernia

Many people who have just been told they have a hiatus hernia worry that such a diagnosis must eventually mean an operation. This anxiety can be dispelled in the vast majority of cases. A combination of the self-management and lifestyle changes discussed in chapter 7 with a simple drug regimen is usually sufficient to keep complications—and the surgeon—at bay.

Antacids

Antacids neutralize acid that has already been produced by the stomach. For many hiatus hernia sufferers, all that is needed is an acceptable antacid that they can take whenever the symptoms arise. They can take as many as they wish, after meals and when they have heartburn. The choice of antacid is the patient's; there are many different remedies to choose from, and the pharmacist is as knowledgeable about them as the doctor.

If something a little longer-acting is needed, you may be prescribed a combination of an antacid with an *alginate*, a medicine derived from seaweed that forms a sticky alkaline barrier against gastric juices. This reduces reflux and helps avoid contact between the acidic stomach juices and the esophagus. Among the alginate-containing compounds (some are combined with antacid, some with H2-antagonists; see below) are Gastrocote and Gaviscon.

A combination of antacid with a silicone (dimethylpolysiloxane, dimethicone, or simethicone) may be used in similar circumstances. The silicone reduces surface tension and acts as a defoaming agent, which is thought to make it easier to belch and to allow more rapid passage of food and digestive juices through the stomach, reducing reflux as it does so. Preparations containing dimethicone include Gas-X, Maalox Anti-Gas, Mylanta Gas Relief, Mylicon Infants' Drops, and Phazyme.

All these preparations are popular over-the-counter drugs, which must mean that they work at least to some extent—but be aware that they have failed to work satisfactorily in good, large-scale trials. What I will say about them here is that if they suit you, you may as well stick with them. However, if you need them every day, you probably should step up your medical treatment to a regimen that has been proven to work. Such a regimen usually includes drugs that suppress acid secretion by the stomach: the H2-antagonists and the proton pump inhibitors.

Acid Suppressants

Acid-suppressant drugs act by stopping the stomach from secreting acid. The first ones introduced were the *H2-antagonists* (also called *H2-blockers*). "H2" stands for *histamine H2-receptor*, which is part of the chemical mechanism used by the stomach for making acid. By blocking it, these drugs greatly reduce acid production. H2-antagonists reduce rather than completely eliminate acid from the stomach—but the reduction is enough to make a very clear difference in the amount of acid refluxing through the cardia and to be of great benefit in esophagitis.

H2-Antagonists

Cimetidine, or Tagamet, was the first H2-antagonist. It revolutionized the treatment of gastric and peptic ulcers. It proved marginally less successful in esophagitis caused by hiatus hernia; in many patients the symptoms, but not the esophagitis (as assessed by endoscopy), decreased. The dose of cimetidine for hiatus hernia ranges from 400 milligrams (mg) four times daily to 800 mg each evening. Patients may find they have to experiment with different doses before settling on what is best for them.

Ranitidine (Zantac) was the second H2-antagonist. It is very similar in effect to cimetidine in relieving symptoms, although one large report suggested that it was more effective than cimetidine in healing esophagitis. A single 300-mg dose in the evening is now preferred (rather than 150 mg twice daily). Patients who do not heal on this dose can be given doses up to 1,500 mg daily (not a dose used often) to get added benefit.

Newer H2-antagonists include famotidine (Pepcid) and niza-tidine (Axid); they seem to be similar to ranitidine and cimetidine, with no particular advantages over them.

Proton Pump Inhibitors

The proton pump is the mechanism by which gastric lining cells produce hydrogen ions (i.e, acid). Proton pump inhibitors block this mechanism so that no acid is produced. Put simply, they act at a stage before H2-antagonists in the chain of chemical processes that finally lead to acid secretion into the stomach. H2-antago-nists do not block all acid production—proton pump inhibitors do.

The first of the proton pump inhibitors was omeprazole (Prilosec in the United States; Losec in Canada). It has recently been joined by a second, lansoprazole (Prevacid). Proton pump inhibitors are much more powerful blockers of stomach secretions than H2-antagonists, so one dose can completely remove all acid from the stomach, and therefore from an irritated esophagus, for a full twenty-four hours. They improve symptoms and heal esophagitis faster than ranitidine or cimetidine.

Separate studies have shown that patients failing to respond to cimetidine or to ranitidine improved on omeprazole. In fact, all the patients who failed to heal on ranitidine healed on omeprazole.

The trials suggest that 90 percent of patients with esophagitis heal on omeprazole treatment, with one dose of either 20 mg or 40 mg daily, given for four to twelve weeks. Lansoprazole is probably as effective as omeprazole, but the clinical evidence for its action is not as comprehensive; omeprazole remains the leading drug in this field.

Given these results, it may be surprising that not everyone with esophagitis is given omeprazole—and I sympathize with this view. However, in these days of cost-consciousness about medical treatment, if everyone with heartburn were given omeprazole, it would greatly increase the immediate costs of health care, possibly to the detriment of other needy groups of patients. Omeprazole still tends, therefore, to be reserved for people who have failed to heal on less expensive treatment (such as careful lifestyle management plus an antacid or an H2-antagonist) or whose severe symptoms obviously need urgent treatment.

Antacids and acid suppressants are not the only choices for people with hiatus hernias and acid reflux; other groups of drugs include the motility enhancers and the mucosal protectors.

Motility Enhancers

Motility enhancers (or *prokinetics*) have three main actions that theoretically should help hiatus hernia sufferers. They improve the efficiency of the muscles in the wall of the esophagus, so that it transfers food into the stomach faster. They speed up the emptying of the stomach, and they increase muscle tone in the sphincter between the esophagus and the stomach. By closing off the barrier between stomach and esophagus, they make it harder for the stomach contents to flow backward up into the esophagus. And by opening the exit from stomach to duodenum, the time when the stomach remains full is shorter, lessening the chance of such backward and upward flow.

Motility enhancers in current use in North America include bethanechol (Duvoid, Urabeth, Urecholine), domperidone (Motil-

ium; available in Canada), and metoclopramide (Octamide, Metoclopramide Intensol, Reglan). On their own, motility enhancers
are rarely a complete treatment, but they can augment the effect
of H2-antagonists and proton pump inhibitors. Side effects of
motility enhancers include drowsiness and diarrhea and a condition called hyperprolactinemia, which can lead to the breast's ooz-
ing a milky fluid, even in men. Long-term treatment with metoclopramide, particularly in older people, can produce *tardive
dyskinesia*, characterized by muscle twitching and uncontrolled
movements such as nervous tics. Domperidone is probably less
likely to cause these effects than metoclopramide.

Mucosal Protectors

Three drugs—carbenoxolone (Bioplex and Pyrogastrone in the
U.K.), sucralfate (Carafate), and tripotassium dicitratobismuthate
(De-Nol in the U.K.)—are known as *mucosal protective agents*.
They are probably more useful against stomach and duodenal
ulcers than against esophagitis, because they are present in the
lower esophagus for too little time to make much difference. They
have no effect on acid production or on gut motility; they appear
to alter the quality of the mucus in the stomach and esophagus so
that it protects the underlying lining cells against acid and pepsin
attack.

Studies have shown that Pyrogastrone (actually a combination of carbenoxolone and an alginate) healed esophageal ulcers
more effectively than an antacid alone and that it was as effective
as cimetidine in reducing symptoms and healing esophagitis.

A drawback to carbenoxolone is that it can cause retention of
salt and water, so it can raise blood pressure in susceptible persons;
care must be taken to check the blood pressure regularly in people
taking the drug for long periods.

Trials of sucralfate have had differing results. One trial showed
it to be no better than a placebo (a dummy tablet) at healing
reflux-induced esophagitis. Others had better success; some

showed it to be as effective as an antacid-alginate combination in reducing symptoms and healing esophagitis, while others showed it to be only slightly less effective than ranitidine or cimetidine. One study found that it helped cases of esophagitis that had failed to respond to cimetidine or ranitidine.

A problem with sucralfate is that it must be given at least two hours before or after other frequently prescribed drugs, such as the antibiotic tetracycline, the anti-epilepsy drug phenytoin, the heart-rate regulator digoxin, and cimetidine. This is because it can interfere with their absorption or metabolism—and therefore possibly alter their effectiveness. People prescribed sucralfate must therefore know exactly how often they must take their drugs and when.

De-Nol is mainly used for gastric and duodenal ulcers, but it is also gaining a reputation for healing esophagitis, although there are no satisfactory and comprehensive trials of it in this area. It is more often used nowadays as part of a package of two or three drugs to eradicate the bacterium *Helicobacter pylori* from the stomach of people with ulcers.

Eradicating Helicobacter

Helicobacter pylori is a bacterium that was first brought to the world's attention in 1982 by Dr. B. J. Marshall, a young hospital physician in Perth, Western Australia. He cultured it from a specimen taken from the stomach of an ulcer patient. The story of how this turned into the scientific detective story of the twentieth century is told in detail in my book *Coping with Stomach Ulcers*. Suffice it to say here that we now know that many stomach and duodenal ulcers are caused by infection with *Helicobacter pylori* and that regimens combining various drugs have been devised to eradicate this bacterium. In this way, the ulcers have been cured and have not recurred—as ulcers do when they heal with H2-antagonists.

On the assumption that *Helicobacter pylori* may also have something to do with reflux-associated esophageal ulcers—and particularly with the esophageal ulcers that occur in Barrett's esophagus—some doctors are using anti-*Helicobacter* regimens to treat people with moderate and severe reflux esophagitis. The jury is still out on the part played by *Helicobacter* in esophageal ulcers, but anti-*Helicobacter* treatment seems to help some patients who are resistant to the mainstream drugs. We have to wait for published trial evidence to be sure one way or the other.

In the meantime, two main anti-*Helicobacter* treatment regimens have been established. One is triple therapy, combining omeprazole or lansoprazole with a week's course of two of the three antibiotics clarithromycin, amoxicillin, and metronidazole. Alternatively, De-Nol is combined with tetracycline and metronidazole. The other is a dual combination of ranitidine bismuth citrate (Pylorid in Canada) with either amoxicillin or clarithromycin. They are highly effective against peptic ulcers in the stomach and duodenum; whether they are as effective against esophagitis remains to be seen.

Anticholinergics

Something must be written here about another group of drugs, the *anticholinergics*. They include dicyclomine, pirenzepine (Gastrozepin in Canada), and propantheline (Pro-Banthine). They were much used in the past because they tended to reduce acid secretion, but at the same time they also slowed down the progress of food through the gut—not an action needed for people with esophagitis! They also introduce a host of uncomfortable side effects, such as blurred vision, constipation, and, in men with enlarged prostate glands, retention of urine. Therefore the anticholinergics are no longer the first choice for any form of acid-ulcer disease, including esophagitis.

Combining Drug Treatments

Many doctors use the belt-and-suspenders principle in treating more severe hiatus hernia symptoms—they prescribe combinations of drugs, rather than single ones. I have great sympathy with their viewpoint and have often done so myself. However, there is little published evidence that combinations are more effective in treating hiatus hernia with esophagitis than, say, omeprazole alone.

Combination studies that have been published cover cimetidine used with alginate, with metoclopramide, and with cisapride. On the whole, they had mixed results, and for scientific proof of benefit, more studies are needed. However, it is difficult to see how such studies can be conducted now that we have moved on to using omeprazole. General practitioners like myself are likely to use a choice of different regimens, tailored to suit each individual patient. This may mean ringing the changes between H2-antagonists and proton pump inhibitors, and adding other drugs where it seems necessary, more convenient for, or more acceptable to the patient.

Most doctors will approach the patient with hiatus hernia and symptoms of esophagitis in roughly the following way:

1. Give advice on general health measures as described in chapter 7 plus antacid tablets for the occasional bout of heartburn. If that does not work, then:

2. Add an H2-antagonist to the antacid regimen, and use this combination for four to six weeks. If that does not work, then:

3. Give omeprazole for up to eight weeks, then review again. This will cure more than 90 percent of cases of esophagitis. If that does not work, then refer to a specialist for further investigation and management.

4. Combinations of omeprazole or an H2-antagonist with motility promoters or mucosal protectors may be tried if there is evidence of, say, motility disorders (such as feel-

ings of fullness and belching) or of painful swallowing (when sucralfate seems particularly effective). Where it remains difficult to control symptoms, and where sur-geons have recommended medical treatment only, then other combinations may be tried—on an empirical basis rather than because any good evidence for them exists.

Mention must be made of drugs that may worsen esophagitis and that must be avoided or taken with extreme care by people with hiatus hernia.

Drugs and Foods to Be Avoided (Or Used with Care)

Some drugs and some foods actually tend to relax the sphincter between the esophagus and the stomach, making reflux easier. These include fats, so fatty meals should be avoided. Other sub-stances that can promote reflux in this way include coffee, choco-late, peppermint, alcohol, and tobacco. The drugs that do so (at least under experimental conditions) include theophylline, used in asthma to relieve wheezing; nitrates (such as nitroglycerine and isosorbide), given to relax the coronary arteries in angina; and the progestogens used as part of the hormone cycle in the contracep-tive pill. As mentioned above, anticholinergic drugs, often given for peptic ulcers, also tend to lead to reflux.

Other drugs that may delay the emptying of the stomach into the duodenum—and that may thus create the conditions for reflux—include bronchodilator drugs (which open the airways), like salbutamol for asthma, and some calcium antagonist drugs used to lower high blood pressure. However, their use for asthma and high blood pressure may be more important than their possi-ble (and unproven) side effects on esophagitis, so they should not be stopped unless they give rise to symptoms or make symptoms worse. This goes for all the drugs and foods mentioned above.

People taking, eating, or drinking them should keep their possible side effects in mind but not necessarily stop them without good reason to do so.

The reasons for referring patients for surgery and a description of the surgical procedures are set forth in the next chapter.

Chapter 9

Surgery for Hiatus Hernia

M aking the decision to operate on a hiatus hernia is not easy. It has been made much less difficult in recent years with the introduction of omeprazole and lansoprazole, because many more people with reflux-induced esophagitis now respond very well to medical treatment. Since failure of medical treatment has always been the main reason for surgery, the effectiveness of these drugs has reduced the numbers needing operations.

However, there still remains a substantial number of sufferers from hiatus hernia for whom surgery is the only answer. Apart from the small number (less than 10 percent) of people who do not find relief from drugs, some younger adults have symptoms that recur as soon as they stop continuous medical treatment. People in this category are often uneasy about taking drugs for years at a time that completely suppress stomach-acid secretion. Some basis for this fear may be legitimate, because a small—though only theoretical—risk exists of the use of these drugs leading to a type of stomach tumor called *gastric carcinoid*. It must be stressed, however, that no rise has been reported in such tumors since omeprazole was launched in the late 1980s, and it has been prescribed to many millions of people for long periods.

Other reasons for surgery include the appearance of complications of severe reflux, such as strictures (causing swallowing difficulties and regurgitation) or Barrett's esophagus (with bleeding, severe pain, or the threat of perforation). Surgery is also indicated where reflux is linked to motility disorders such as achalasia or nutcracker esophagus and in children who have not responded to the postural therapy described in chapters 1 and 3. Some people develop reflux disease only after a previous stomach operation for a severe peptic ulcer; they too need surgery rather than medical treatment.

Finally, a small group of people (around 4 percent of all people with a hiatus hernia) exists whose symptoms are not caused by reflux of acid, but by the bulk of a rolling hernia in the chest. For many of them, surgery is the only way of reducing their very distressing symptoms.

Here I must say how grateful I am to the work and the publications of Professor Alfred Cuschieri, of the University of Dundee. I am not a surgeon, so this chapter reviewing surgical treatment of hiatus hernia has necessarily been drawn from his huge background of knowledge and experience. In his book *Reflux Oesophagitis* (written with Drs. T. P. J. Hennessy and J. R. Bennett), he admits that the ideal operation has yet to be established. There are many different operations, and each one has its share of postoperative complications.

Surgery for hiatus hernia has two main aims:

1. To return the hernia from above the diaphragm to its proper abdominal site and to close the hiatus around the esophagus so that this material cannot return to the chest cavity. This is the diaphragmatic repair.

2. To reshape the junction between the stomach and the lower end of the esophagus (the cardia) to make sure that any reflux is minimized. The usual way to do this is through a procedure called *fundoplication*, in which part of the fundus is wrapped around the last two inches of the esophagus and stitched in place.

The Choice of Operation

Since the diaphragm lies between the chest and abdomen, it can be approached either from below, through the abdomen, or from above, through the chest. For most people with a relatively uncomplicated hiatus hernia, an abdominal operation is chosen. The choice of route, however, depends partly on the patient's build. If the hiatus is set deeply inside the abdomen and the angle between the lower ribs (at the lower end of the breastbone) is narrow, or if the patient is overweight, the surgeon may prefer to go through the chest. This is the easier route in such patients, and it has also proved both safer and to result in a better outcome for them.

The surgeon may also go through the chest if the patient has undergone previous abdominal surgery (perhaps on the stomach or gallbladder) or if the esophagus is shorter than normal (usually due to scarring from years of esophagitis). In some people with a large rolling hernia, the surgeon may decide to open both chest and abdomen.

Recently, *laparoscopic* surgery has been developed, in which the repair is done through a flexible tube, just like the endoscopy tube, that is inserted into the abdomen, leaving a minimal scar. It is only suitable for a small group of patients with less severe reflux problems, and it must be carried out by a very experienced surgeon.

Many different operations exist for hiatus hernia, often named after the surgeon who invented a particular technique. The most common abdominal approach is to wrap the fundus around three-quarters of the lowest five centimeters (two inches) of the esophagus, stitch the wrap in place, and stitch the outside surface of the wrap to the left crural muscle on the lower surface of the diaphragm. This fulfils the two purposes of creating a better one-way valve between esophagus and stomach and of fixing the junction firmly in place under the diaphragm (see Figure 9.1). It also appears to result in the fewest and least severe postoperative complications.

With the approach through the chest, the technique most preferred is called the Belsey Mark IV operation. It involves wrapping and stitching the fundus twice around the front of the lower esophagus and returning the hernia below the diaphragm, where the hiatus is repaired and the outer "wrap" is stitched to the crural muscle, anchoring it there. With a smaller and tighter hiatus and the esophageal-stomach junction firmly fixed under the diaphragm, there is little chance of recurrence.

The Short Esophagus

For some people, the routine operation is not enough, because the esophagus is too short for its lower end to be brought without tension into the abdomen. This condition, known as *short esophagus*, can be a complication caused by long-standing esophagitis or by previous operations for hiatus hernia, or it may be the result of an inherited short esophagus from childhood.

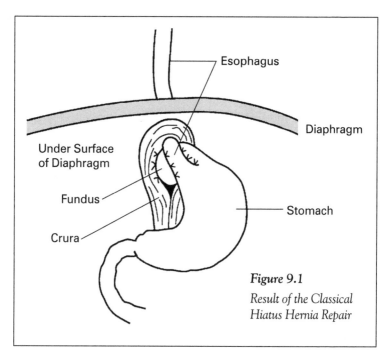

Figure 9.1

Result of the Classical Hiatus Hernia Repair

Surgery for short esophagus is best carried out in a hospital unit specializing in esophageal complications. In one such operation (the Collis-Nissen operation) the esophagus is lengthened by refashioning part of the upper stomach to turn it into a replacement lower esophagus. In another, a length of bowel is used.

In children, surgery is delayed until after the second birthday, because more than 80 percent of children born with a hiatus hernia respond perfectly well to medical management alone, and the hernia disappears by age two. The preferred operation for most youngsters whose symptoms continue after the second birthday is a complete fundal wrap around the whole lower esophagus, which is then stitched to the underside of the diaphragm. Children differ from adults in that they must be tube-fed through the abdominal wall for a short time after surgery, to allow the stomach, diaphragm, and esophagus to heal.

Strictures and Bougies

A major complication of long-standing esophagitis is stricture: a rigid narrowing of the lower esophagus due to fibrous scarring. Strictures cause difficulties in swallowing when the inside diameter of the esophagus shrinks to below 12 millimeters (about half an inch). At this level, such strictures can be relatively easily treated with medical treatment and bouginage (see below). A stricture less than three millimeters in diameter and more than 3 centimeters long proves the existence of serious esophageal disease that will probably need more-extensive surgery. The higher up the esophagus a stricture is found, the more likely it is to be caused by Barrett's esophagus, with all the extra risks this diagnosis entails.

The main symptom of a stricture is difficulty in swallowing. At first this is an occasional embarrassment; later (months or even years later in adults; it progresses faster in children) it becomes more constant. It is eventually linked with loss of weight and sometimes bleeding and anemia. Regurgitation from food stuck above the stricture can lead to chest infections.

After X-rays and endoscopy have established the diagnosis, the usual initial treatment is to try to open up the stricture by *bouginage*. This involves passing metal, spindle-shaped *bougies* (solid structures not unlike tiny torpedoes) over a guide wire inserted down through the stricture by means of an endoscope. The procedure starts with a small bougie, which is replaced by larger and larger bougies until the stricture is stretched to an adequate diameter.

This operation may sound horrific, but the patient is well prepared beforehand with an injection of a tranquilizer into a vein and a local anesthetic into the throat. Very nervous patients are offered a general anesthetic, although this is rarely needed. People can usually swallow normally if the stricture diameter is increased to 15 millimeters. If a stricture is very rigid and resists dilation, a second session may be needed some days later.

Some people require a series of dilations before they can swallow satisfactorily. Those who still have trouble after three months of repeat dilations probably need surgery, provided they are generally fit for it.

Simply removing the stricture does not remove the cause of the stricture—which is usually esophagitis due to acid reflux—so constant medical treatment for such esophagitis is mandatory to prevent recurrence. As a last resort, the only way to prevent recurrence may be surgical repair of the hiatus hernia and the reflux.

Postscript

Perhaps the last words on hiatus hernia and esophagitis should be left to a real expert in the disease, Professor Alfred Cuschieri. In the preface to his book *Reflux Oesophagitis*, intended for medical professionals, he wrote that the outcomes of recent research efforts include a better appreciation of the nature of esophagitis and more effective drugs for its control. He also stated that the complex relationships between reflux disease, motility disorders, abnormal circulation in the gut, and chest pain are now being unraveled. There is a growing realization, he added, that specialist treatment of the complications of esophageal reflux disease is necessary if such complications are to decline and patients are to benefit.

Professor Cuschieri's book—and his other publications on reflux disease and hiatus hernia—provide the solid framework upon which general practitioners like myself, faced daily with patients suffering from the symptoms of hiatus hernia and esophagitis, base our treatments. I hope that *Positive Options for Hiatus Hernia* contributes by giving readers some idea of the modern expert's approach to managing a hiatus hernia without losing too many readers in technicalities.

My aim was neither to frighten readers about, nor to gloss over, the problems produced by a hiatus hernia, but to inform sufferers and their families about its modern management. It was also to translate into layman's language the knowledge I have gained in practice from treating patients and from reading the work of experts like Professor Cuschieri and his academic and surgical colleagues. As we medical professionals grow ever more aware of the need to keep our patients closely informed about the details of their disorders, the possible treatments, and their likely outcomes, it seems such books are needed. I hope this one has achieved its aims. Thank you for reading it.

Glossary of Medical Terms

achalasia — Spasm of the esophagus, leading to difficulties in swallowing.

acid suppressants — Drugs that stop the stomach from producing acid.

alginate — Seaweed-derived material that forms a foam, which protects the esophagus from acid attack.

anemia — A deficiency of red blood cells, leading to poor oxygen supply to the body.

angina pectoris—Chest pain that falls short of a full heart attack.

antacids — Drugs that neutralize acids formed by the stomach.

anticholinergics — A group of drugs used commonly in the past that tend to reduce acid secretion.

antispasmodic drugs — Drugs that prevent muscle spasm and that slow peristalsis.

aorta / inferior vena cava — The main blood vessels from and to the heart. They pass through the diaphragm.

autonomic nervous system — Controls the movements of food from the pharynx through the rest of the gut, without our being aware of it.

backflow — A condition in which material inside the gut passes upward toward the mouth, rather than downward away from the mouth.

bacterium — A germ that may cause infection (such as *Helicobacter*).

barium-swallow — An X-ray technique to show how the esophagus and diaphragm are working.

Barrett's esophagus — (also called Barrett's syndrome) A condition in which the lowest region of the esophagus is much more prone than normal to ulceration.

bile — The green, bitter juice produced by the liver and concentrated in the gallbladder.

biopsy — The taking of a piece of tissue for examination.

bougie — An instrument designed to pass through and open up (dilate) a stricture, or a narrowing, in the esophagus.

cardia — The junction between the esophagus and the stomach.

catheter — A fine, hollow tube usually used to drain fluids from the stomach.

crura — The arrangement of crossed muscles that helps to hold the lower esophagus in place under the diaphragm.

crural muscle — The muscle within the crura.

diaphragm — The broad sheet of muscle separating the chest from the abdomen.

diaphragmatic crura — Powerful muscles in the hiatus's rim that hold it close to the esophagus and make sure nothing can slip upward from the abdomen into the chest cavity through the hiatus.

diffuse spasm — A spasm that spreads all along the length of the esophagus.

dilation — The widening or opening up of a tube, such as the esophagus.

duodenum — The first part of the small bowel, just after the stomach.

dysphagia — Difficulty in swallowing.

endoscopy — The act of looking into an organ with a flexible fiber-optic tube.

esophagitis — Inflammation of the esophagus.

esophagus — The gullet, or passage that moves food from the throat to the stomach; it lies mainly in the chest.

fundus — The top 10 percent of the stomach, which lies above the cardia.

fundoplication — A procedure in which part of the fundus is wrapped around the last two inches of the esophagus and stitched in place.

gastric carcinoid — A type of stomach tumor.

gastric juices — The acid and pepsin juices produced by the stomach to start digestion.

gastritis — Inflammation of the stomach.

gastroenterology — The study of the digestive system.

gastroesophageal sphincter — A ring of muscle within the wall of the cardia, just where the esophagus becomes the stomach. It controls the passage of food and food residues from one segment of the digestive tract to the next and prevents backflow.

H2-antagonists — (also called H2 blockers) Acid-suppressant drugs that act by stopping the secretion of acid by the stomach.

hemoglobin — The oxygen-carrying pigment in red blood cells.

hemorrhage — Severe bleeding.

hernia — The projection of a piece of gut into a space outside the abdomen.

hernial sac — The "bag" of membrane in which a hernia lies.

herniation — The moment at which a hernia occurs.

hiatus — The hole in the diaphragm through which the lower esophagus passes.

laparoscopic tube — A flexible endoscope through which surgeons operate inside the abdomen; it is passed through the abdominal wall.

larynx — The voice box, situated at the junction between the pharynx and the esophagus.

manometry — The measurement of pressure inside a hollow tube.

melena — The passing of black blood in the stools.

motility — The normal movement of the muscles in the walls of the esophagus, stomach, and the rest of the gut.

motility enhancers — (also called prokinetics) Drugs that improve the efficiency of the muscles in the wall of the esophagus; speed up the emptying of the stomach; close off the barrier between stomach and esophagus; and open the exit from stomach to duodenum.

mucosal protective agents — Drugs that appear to alter the quality of the mucus in the stomach and esophagus so that it protects the underlying lining cells against acid and pepsin attack.

nutcracker esophagus — A painful condition in the chest in which the sufferer is aware of strong contractions of the esophageal muscle.

oblique muscles — Muscles that run at an angle in the gut wall, rather than along it or around it. They keep the angle between esophagus and stomach precisely correct.

paraesophageal hernia — A hernia (usually of the fundus) that comes through the diaphragm alongside the esophagus.

pepsin — A juice produced by the stomach to start to digest proteins.

perforation — A hole through the wall of the esophagus or stomach caused by an ulcer.

peristalsis — The normal wave of muscle contraction that pushes food onward during digestion; normal peristalsis gives normal motility.

pharynx — The back of the throat, between mouth and larynx.

placebo — A dummy tablet with no effect, used as a comparison with new treatments to assess their effects.

postural therapy — Treatment for healing the esophagus by keeping the patient upright or in a particular body position.

pyloric stenosis — In children, a benign overgrowth of muscle tissue around the outlet of the stomach into the duodenum. In adults, a narrowing of the pylorus due to scarring from long-term ulceration.

reflux — Backflow of stomach contents upwards into the esophagus.

regimen — The overall treatment advised for a patient.

regurgitation — The bringing of swallowed food back into the mouth.

retrosternal pain — Pain behind the breastbone, presumed to come from the heart until proved otherwise.

short esophagus — A condition in which the esophagus is too short for its lower end to be brought without tension into the abdomen.

spasm — A form of muscle cramp, e.g., in the esophagus.

sphincter — A ring of muscle around particular areas of the gut (the cardia, the stomach-duodenum junction, the small bowel-large bowel junction, and the anus); when active it stops food from passing backward and impels it onward.

stricture — A ringlike piece of scar tissue that narrows the gut and can lead to complete blockage if not relieved.

tardive dyskinesia — A condition characterized by muscle twitching and uncontrolled movements such as nervous tics and often caused by long-term treatment with metoclopramide.

tertiary contractions — A form of peristalsis whose purpose seems to be to churn food rather than pass it on; tertiary contractions cannot be felt.

tracheoesophageal atresia — A blind end on the esophagus that does not meet up with the stomach at all.

tracheoesophageal fistulae — Abnormal open connections between the esophagus and the breathing system.

ulcer — A raw, punched-out area in the lining of the esophagus, stomach, or duodenum caused by acid and/or pepsin and the loss of the natural protection against them.

waterbrash — A sour or bitter watery fluid that appears without warning in the mouth; a sign of regurgitation from the stomach.

Index

Index

POSITIVE OPTIONS FOR CROHN'S DISEASE: Self-Help and Treatment by Joan Gomez, M.D.

Crohn's Disease is an inflammatory bowel disease that, while non-fatal, can be devastating and is spreading at an increasing rate in Western countries. This book provides information about the digestive system, causes and symptoms of Crohn's disease, who is at risk and why, diagnostic methods, and new, exciting treatment research—all written in clear and simple language.

Recommendations for managing the disease are accompanied by detailed self-help options. Dietary changes are key, from creating an optimal personal diet to boosting the immune system with special foods. An important chapter addresses lifestyle choices that can alleviate the depression and anxiety that may accompany this traumatic and sometimes embarassing illness.

192 pages...Paperback...$12.95... Hardcover... $22.95

CHINESE HERBAL MEDICINE MADE EASY: Natural and Effective Remedies for Common Illnesses
by Thomas Richard Joiner

Chinese herbal medicine is an ancient system for maintaining health and prolonging life. This book demystifies the subject, with clear explanations and easy-to-read alphabetical listings of more than 750 herbal remedies for over 250 common illnesses ranging from acid reflux and AIDS to breast cancer, pain management, sexual dysfunction, and weight loss. Whether you are a newcomer to herbology or a seasoned practitioner, you will find this book a valuable addition to your health library.

448 pages...Paperback...$24.95... Hardcover... $34.95

FAD-FREE NUTRITION *by* Frederick J. Stare, M.D., Ph.D., and Elizabeth M. Whelan, Sc.D, M.P.H.

From the American Council on Science and Health, a no-nonsense book that challenges trendy diets and offers sound information about how to eat normally and eat right. From explaining why the produce at the supermarket is indeed safe, to describing which foods can boost immune system functioning, to showing how easy the food pyramid really is, this book puts the joy back into food.

256 pages ... Paperback $14.95

To order books see last page or call (800) 266-5592

CANCER—INCREASING YOUR ODDS FOR SURVIVAL: A Resource Guide for Integrating Mainstream, Alternative and Complementary Therapies *by* David Bognar

Based on the four-part television series hosted by Walter Cronkite, this book provides a comprehensive look at traditional medical treatments for cancer and how they can be supplemented. It explains the basics of cancer and the best actions to take immediately after a diagnosis of cancer. It outlines the various conventional, alternative, and complementary treatments; describes the powerful effect the mind can have on the body and the therapies that strengthen this connection; and explores the spiritual healing and issues surrounding death and dying.

Includes full-length interviews with leaders in the field of healing, including Joan Borysenko, Stephen Levine, and Bernie Siegel.

352 pages ... Paperback $15.95 ... Hardcover $25.95

CANCER DOESN'T HAVE TO HURT: How to Conquer the Pain Caused by Cancer and Cancer Treatment
by Pamela J. Haylock, R.N., and Carol P. Curtiss, R.N.

Studies have shown that people with cancer benefit by taking control over the treatment of the disease and their pain. Written with warmth and clarity by two oncology nurses with more than 50 years of experience between them, this guide explains cancer pain, explores the emotional effects on sufferers and caregivers, and shows readers how to manage pain using a combination of medical and natural self-help treatments. Includes a "Self-Care Workbook " section.

192 pages ... 10 illus. ... Paperback ... $14.95 ... Hardcover $24.95

HOW WOMEN CAN FINALLY STOP SMOKING
by Robert C. Klesges, Ph.D., and Margaret DeBon

This guide reveals that what works for men does not necessarily work for women when quitting smoking. Women tend to gain more weight, their menstrual cycles and menopause affect the likelihood of success, and their withdrawal symptoms are different.

Part One guides women in choosing the best time to quit and in deciding which method to use. *Part Two* gives directions for managing withdrawal and weight gain, finding peer support, and controlling stress.

192 pages ... 3 illus. ... Paperback ... $11.95.

THE COMPLETE GUIDE TO JOSEPH H. PILATES' TECHNIQUES OF PHYSICAL CONDITIONING: Applying the Principles of Body Control
by Allan Menezes, Founder of the Pilates Institute of Australasia

This comprehensive book includes a complete floor program (no special equipment needed) that guides readers through basic, intermediate, and advanced routines, with detailed descriptions of each exercise and step-by-step photographs. There is a special section on relieving back, ankle, and shoulder pain, and insights on how the work can be adapted by athletes. Worksheets are provided to record progress, and an introduction gives the history and legacy of Joseph Pilates.

208 pages ... 191 b/w photos ... 80 illus. & charts ... Paperback $19.95 ... Spiral Bound $26.95

GET FIT WHILE YOU SIT: Easy Workouts from Your Chair
by Charlene Torkelson

Here is a total-body workout that can be done right from your chair, anywhere. It is perfect for office workers, travelers, and those with age-related movement limitations or special conditions. This book offers three programs. The *One-Hour Chair Program* is a full-body, low-impact workout that includes light aerobics and exercises to be done with or without weights. The *5-Day Short Program* features five compact workouts for those short on time. Finally, the *Ten-Minute Miracles* is a group of easy-to-do exercises perfect for anyone on the go.

160 pages ... 212 b/w photos ... Paperback ... $12.95 ... Hardcover $22.95

PEAK PERFORMANCE FITNESS: Maximizing Your Fitness Potential Without Injury or Strain
by Jennifer Rhodes, M.S.PT. Foreword by Joan E. Edelstein

Jennifer Rhodes looks at the body as an integrated system and offers a step-by-step plan for developing cardiovascular capacity, strength, and flexibility based on your body type and posture. She gives real-life success stories of how her approach has helped clients, while detailed photographs and anatomical drawings illustrate the exercises. If you are serious about long-term health and want to get to your best body ever, this book will help you redefine the way you exercise and move.

160 pages ... 46 b/w photos ... 31 illus...Paperback ... $14.95

ALZHEIMER'S EARLY STAGES: First Steps in Caring and Treatment *by* Daniel Kuhn, MSW

This book is for the family and friends of those recently diagnosed with Alzheimer's. The first part discusses how the disease affects the brain, known risk factors, the latest treatments, and guidelines for prevention. An important chapter presents what it is like to live with Alzheimer's.

Part Two covers changing relationships, developing new lines of communication, taking responsibility for decisions, and encouraging the patient to try to slow the progress of the disease. Kuhn recommends starting long-term planning immediately and addresses ways that caregivers should take care of themselves.

288 pages ... Paperback $14.95 ... Hardcover $24.95

ALTERNATIVE TREATMENTS FOR FIBROMYALGIA AND CHRONIC FATIGUE SYNDROME: Insights from Practitioners and Patients *by* Mari Skelly and Andrea Helm; Foreword by Paul Brown, M.D., Ph.D.

Many people suffering from fibromyalgia and CFS are unable to find effective treatment and relief. This book combines interviews with practitioners of alternative therapies—including acupuncture, massage therapy, chiropractic, psychotherapy, and energetic healing—with personal stories from patients. These offer a firsthand look at symptoms, treatments, struggles and successes, lifestyle adaptations and medicine, diet, and activity regimens that might help others. There are also sections on obtaining health insurance and Social Security disability.

288 pages ... Paperback... $15.95 ... Hardcover... $25.95

CHRONIC FATIGUE SYNDROME, FIBROMYALGIA, AND OTHER INVISIBLE ILLNESSES: A Comprehensive and Compassionate Guide *by* Katrina Berne, Ph.D.

A new edition of the classic work *Running on Empty,* this greatly revised and expanded book has the latest findings on chronic fatigue syndrome and comprehensive information about fibromyalgia, a related condition. Overlapping diseases such as environmental illness, breast implant inflammatory syndrome, lupus, Sjogren's syndrome, and post-polio syndrome are also discussed. The book includes possible causes, symptoms, diagnostic processes, and options for treatment

352 pages ... Paperback... $15.95 ... Hardcover... $25.95

All prices subject to change

MENOPAUSE WITHOUT MEDICINE
by Linda Ojeda, Ph.D. ... New Fourth Edition

Linda Ojeda broke new ground 15 years ago with this bestselling resource on menopause, giving women a clear understanding of menopausal changes and guidelines for effective self-care.

In this new edition she re-examines the hormone therapy debate; suggests natural remedies for depression, hot flashes, sexual changes, and skin and hair problems; and presents an illustrated basic exercise program. She also includes up-to-date information on natural sources of estrogen, including phytoestrogens, and how diet and personality affect mood swings.

352 pages ... 32 illus. ... 62 tables ... Paperback $15.95... Hardcover $25.95

THE NATURAL ESTROGEN DIET: Healthy Recipes for Perimenopause and Menopause
by Dr. Lana Liew with Linda Ojeda, Ph.D.

Two women's health and nutrition experts offer women almost 100 easy and delicious recipes to naturally increase their level of estrogen. Each recipe includes nutritional information such as the calories, cholesterol, and calcium content. The authors also provide an overview of how estrogen can be derived from the food we eat, describe which foods are the highest in estrogen content, and offer meal plan ideas.

224 pages ... 25 illus. ... Paperback ... $13.95

HER HEALTHY HEART: A Woman's Guide to Preventing and Reversing Heart Disease Naturally
by Linda Ojeda, Ph.D.

Almost twice as many women die from heart disease and stroke as from all forms of cancer combined. In fact, heart disease is the #1 killer of American women ages 44 to 65, yet until now most of the research and attention has been given to men. This book fills this gap by addressing the unique aspects of heart disease in women and the natural ways to combat it. Dr. Ojeda explains how women can prevent heart disease whether they take hormone replacement therapy (HRT) or not. She provides detailed information on how to reduce the risk of heart disease through diet, physical activity, and stress management.

352 pages ... Paperback $14.95 ... Hardcover $24.95

To order books see last page or call (800) 266-5592

ORDER FORM

10% DISCOUNT on orders of $50 or more —
20% DISCOUNT on orders of $150 or more —
30% DISCOUNT on orders of $500 or more —
On cost of books for fully prepaid orders

NAME

ADDRESS

CITY/STATE   ZIP/POSTCODE

PHONE   COUNTRY (outside of U.S.)

TITLE	QTY	PRICE	TOTAL
Positive Options ... Hiatus Hernia (paper)		@ $12.95	
Positive Options ... Hiatus Hernia (cloth)		@ $22.95	

Prices subject to change without notice

Please list other titles below:

		@ $	
		@ $	
		@ $	
		@ $	
		@ $	
		@ $	
		@ $	

Check here to receive our book catalog   ☐   FREE

Shipping Costs

First book: $3.00 by bookpost, $4.50 by UPS, Priority Mail, or to ship outside the U.S. Each additional book: $1.00
For rush orders and bulk shipments call us at (800) 266-5592

TOTAL		_____
Less discount @____%		(_____)
TOTAL COST OF BOOKS		_____
Calif. residents add sales tax		_____
Shipping & handling		_____
TOTAL ENCLOSED		_____

Please pay in U.S. funds only

☐ Check ☐ Money Order ☐ Visa ☐ MasterCard ☐ Discover

Card # _____ Exp. date _____

Signature _____

Complete and mail to:
Hunter House Inc., Publishers
PO Box 2914, Alameda CA 94501-0914
Website: www.hunterhouse.com
Orders: (800) 266-5592 or email: ordering@hunterhouse.com
Phone (510) 865-5282 Fax (510) 865-4295

POH 1/01